Transvaginal Sonography
A Clinical Atlas

Transvaginal Sonography
A Clinical Atlas

Arthur C. Fleischer, MD

Professor of Radiology and Radiological Sciences
Associate Professor of Obstetrics and Gynecology
Chief, Diagnostic Sonography
Vanderbilt University Medical Center
Nashville, Tennessee

Donna M. Kepple, RDMS

Chief Sonographer
Vanderbilt University Medical Center
Nashville, Tennessee

With Seven Contributors

J. B. LIPPINCOTT COMPANY   **Philadelphia**
London   New York   Hagerstown

Acquisitions Editor: Lisa McAllister
Sponsoring Editor: Paula Callaghan
Production Manager: Janet Greenwood
Production Coordinator: P. M. Gordon Associates
Compositor: Monotype Composition
Printer/Binder: Arcata Graphics, Halliday
Cover Illustration: Ellen Zink
Cover Design: Louis Fuiano

1 3 5 6 4 2

Library of Congress Cataloging-in-Publication Data

Fleischer, Arthur C.
   Transvaginal sonography : a clinical atlas / Arthur C. Fleischer,
Donna M. Kepple ; with seven contributors.
     p. cm.
   Includes bibliographical references and index.
   ISBN 0-397-51136-1
   1. Ultrasonics in obstetrics—Atlases. 2. Generative organs,
Female—Diseases—Diagnosis—Atlases. 3. Obstetrics—Diagnosis—
Atlases. I. Kepple, Donna M. II. Title.
   [DNLM: 1. Genital Diseases, Female—ultrasonography—atlases.
2. Prenatal Diagnosis—methods—atlases. WP 17 F596t]
RG527.5.U48F54 1992
618′.0457543—dc20
DNLM/DLC
for Library of Congress
                                       91–17424
                                        CIP

To our mothers, who taught us to be caring individuals, and to our families, who allow us time to perfect our thoughts, for as Benjamin Disraeli said in 1877, "The health of the people is really the foundation upon which all their happiness and all their powers as a state depend."

Contributors

Patricia C. Freeman, RT, RDMS

Staff Sonographer
Vanderbilt University Medical Center
Nashville, Tennessee

Philippe Jeanty, MD, PhD

Associate Professor of Radiology and
    Obstetrics and Gynecology
Vanderbilt University Medical Center
Nashville, Tennessee

Bernadette Keefe, MD

Assistant Professor of Radiology and
    Obstetrics and Gynecology
University of North Carolina School of Medicine
Chapel Hill, North Carolina

Charles Odwin, RT, RDMS

Bronx Lebanon Hospital
Bronx, New York

Ronald R. Price, PhD

Professor and Director
Radiological Sciences
Vanderbilt University Medical Center
Nashville, Tennessee

Martin Quinn, MBChB

University of Bristol School of Medicine
Bristol, United Kingdom

Bhaskara K. Rao, MD

Assistant Professor of Radiology
Vanderbilt University Medical Center
Nashville, Tennessee

Preface

Transvaginal sonography (TVS) has greatly enhanced sonographic visualization of pelvic structures. As this clinical atlas demonstrates, major improvements in sonographic diagnosis brought about by TVS have occurred in definitive diagnosis of ectopic pregnancy and evaluation of adnexal masses, as well as detailed depiction of endometrial and myometrial disorders, and early embryonic anatomy.

The purpose of this clinical atlas is to familiarize the reader with the typical sonographic appearances of a variety of disorders. This is done by displaying the native image, without annotations that may distort it, next to a line drawing to draw attention to the areas that need to be noted as well as a line drawing demonstrating the scanning plane in which the image is obtained. When available, the image is compared with the gross pathology, thus enhancing the reader's comprehension of the correlation of the sonographic features with the actual specimen.

The text also includes short chapters on new and specialized applications of TVS such as evaluation of the lower urinary tract and cervix, and the use of transperineal and/or transrectal sonography in a variety of obstetric and gynecologic disorders. The preliminary experience with color Doppler sonography obtained with a transvaginal probe is also discussed.

The reader can refer to this clinical atlas for familiarization with the expected sonographic findings in a particular abnormality. Thus, we hope it is a useful guide for sonographers and sonologists who perform transvaginal sonography.

A. C. F.
D. M. K.

Acknowledgments

We gratefully acknowledge the efforts of several people who greatly assisted in the preparation of this atlas. They include the expert editorial skills of Connie Dehghani, the photography of John Bobbitt, and the artistic skills of Ellen Zink and Charles Odwin, RDMS. We also would like to thank the members of the J. B. Lippincott staff whose expertise and encouragement were appreciated. They include Dean Manke, Lisa McAllister, and the staff in the production department.

We are also grateful to the commercial companies who allowed us to use their equipment both in commercial and prototype form, namely Toshiba America Medical Systems and Siemens, Inc. We thank our departmental chairman, Dr. A. Everette James, Jr., for giving us the opportunity and environment to use this new technique and the facilities to compile this atlas.

Contents

Chapter 1

Instrumentation Used in Transvaginal and Transrectal Sonography

Ronald R. Price, PhD
Arthur C. Fleischer, MD

Introduction

Transvaginal sonography is a recent innovation that requires knowledge of pelvic anatomy, clinical obstetrics and gynecology, and the instrumentation used to obtain diagnostic images. This chapter will discuss the instrumentation used in transvaginal and transrectal sonography.

Improvements in sonographic (ultrasound) instrumentation have primarily resulted from more complete integration of high-speed digital electronics. Special-purpose microcomputers are being used to steer and dynamically focus array transducers, allowing greater flexibility and control over image formation and producing images with both higher spatial and intensity resolution. Recent developments in real-time color Doppler systems have also been the product of high-speed special-purpose microprocessors.

Selection of a satisfactory ultrasound system from the variety of equipment available can often be puzzling and time consuming. It is difficult to obtain an unbiased opinion. Although there are no definite guidelines, there are general considerations.

It is important to understand the principles of ultrasound and to have a fundamental knowledge of how the image is formed. This chapter will review these concepts and each of the categories of transvaginal and transrectal systems, describe the relative advantages and disadvantages of each, and discuss recent advances in each design. In addition, the features of various transducer-probes relative to their clinical use will be emphasized.

Scanner Characteristics

Real-time instruments rapidly sweep the ultrasound beam through a sector, rectangular, or trapezoidal area by either mechanical or electronic means. Frame rates greater than 15 frames per second are required to produce flicker-free images and to observe moving structures. Because real-time probes are not attached to an articulated scanning arm, the sonographer has great flexibility in selecting the image plane orientation.

Ultrasound scanning systems typically consist of:

1. A mechanical or electronic means of moving the ultrasound beam through an image plane;
2. An electronic signal processing unit with controls for varying the transducer power output, overall receiver gain, and other operational parameters such as time-gain compensation (TGC);
3. A gray scan display unit equipped with controls for varying the image brightness and contrast; and
4. A device for permanently recording the images (Polaroid, multi-image format camera, paper prints, videotape, or disk).

The console also has a keyboard to superimpose patient identification, examination date, and study information on the recorded image.

Transducer Designs

Transducers are characterized by their frequency, size (effective aperture in the case of arrays), and degree of focusing. The typical range of frequency for diagnostic ultrasound imaging is 3.5 to 10.0 MHz. The degree of focusing is either short (1 to 4 cm), medium (4 to 8 cm), or long (6 to 12 cm). Focusing is achieved internally by the crystal shape, externally by an acoustic lens, electronically by selective pulsing of individual elements of an array, or by a combination of these three methods. The length of the zone available for focusing (Fresnel zone) is governed by the effective transducer aperture and its operating frequency. In selecting a transducer that has the optimum combination of frequency, aperture size, and focal zone for a particular type of examination, the following points should be considered:

1. Increasing transducer frequency generally results in enhanced axial resolution at the expense of reduced tissue penetration. The highest frequency consistent with adequate tissue penetration should be used.
2. For a selected transducer frequency, decreasing the transducer aperture improves lateral resolution in the near field. The length of the Fresnel zone (useful working range of the transducer) is reduced, however, and lateral resolution beyond this zone (the Fraunhaufer zone) is degraded because of beam divergence. Decreasing the transducer aperture also decreases its sensitivity. It is important to note that many new array systems provide the capability of dynamic aperture, meaning that the effective aperture size can be varied by using smaller or larger subunit transducers depending on the depth of focus chosen.
3. Larger aperture transducers are more suited to lower frequencies to preserve good lateral resolution at depth, whereas smaller apertures are better suited to higher frequency transducers to provide improved lateral resolution over the shorter range. The transvaginal probe is limited because of the size of the transducer contact area, or footprint, relative to anatomic constraints, however.
4. Focused transducers provide improved lateral resolution and sensitivity at the depth of the focal zone, which is limited by the length of the Fresnel zone. The choice of focal zone, therefore, depends on the depth of structures to be resolved.

Alternatives in Scanner Design

The evolution of real-time scanners has led to development of a variety of real-time equipment designs and configurations. It is generally true that no single design provides maximum performance of all imaging parameters; rather, they optimize some imaging parameters at the expense of others. Examples of these are the trade-off of axial resolution obtained from higher frequencies with loss of penetration; good lateral resolution at a specific depth resulting from a large-aperture transducer with decreased lateral resolution at other depths; the convenience of fully electronic scanners against less expensive mechanical scanners; and the large echo-dynamic range of mechanically driven single-element transducers against the more rapid multi-element arrays, which may have a more limited echo-dynamic range. Real-time scanners can be grouped according to how they form the beam (focusing) and how the beam is steered (directed) to form the image. In each case (focusing and steering) the task may be accomplished either mechanically or electronically. The use of acoustic lenses is frequently called mechanical focusing. Single-element transducers use mechanical means exclusively for beam focusing, whereas multi-element arrays use pulse timing to bring about a convergent beam in the plane of the array and use mechanical means to converge the beam in the "slice-thickness" direction (perpendicular to the array axis). Beam steering can be accomplished either by mechanically moving the transducer (or alternatively an acoustic mirror), or by electronic steering by means of pulse-timing sequences in multi-element systems. Hybrid systems are also available that use a combination of array focusing and mechanical steering.

New advances in real-time ultrasonic imaging are largely the result of more complete integration of high-speed dedicated digital electronics (computers) into the imaging systems. The term computed sonography is used to emphasize this increased dependence of the ultrasound image formation on the digital computer.

SINGLE-ELEMENT MECHANICALLY STEERED SCANNERS

Most single-element mechanically steered scanners produce a sector (pie-shaped) format image. The sector opening angles may range from 30 to 120 degrees. Most are approximately 90 degrees.

Mechanically steered scanners have two main advantages relative to electronically steered scanners. First, the use of a single-element transducer requires less sophisticated electronics and generally allows for a more simple transducer head design. Second, there are fewer image artifacts caused by side lobes and grating lobes (unique to electronically steered beams).

There are several disadvantages of mechanically steered arrays. First, the beam focus and beam pattern are fixed for a given transducer. To change the focus, one must change the entire transducer. Second, the image framing rate depends in part on how rapidly the transducer is oscillated. The framing rate is governed by the line density needed to produce an image of diagnostic quality and the depth of the field of view. The velocity of ultrasound in tissue is the ultimate factor governing the oscillation rate of the transducer. The framing rate may become low when large fields of view that require large excursions of the transducer element are chosen. Finally, field-of-view and image frame rates compete in sector format images when the total number of scan lines per image is kept constant. Thus, large opening angles are needed for large field sizes and small opening angles are required for high resolution. In other words, the sector angle must decrease if higher line density is desired. This problem is not unique to mechanical scanners, however, and will be discussed again in relation to electronically steered scanners.

Although many variations on the mechanical oscillating transducer design have been designed and built, the most common design is a transducer that oscillates around a single fixed point and yields a sector-shaped image format (Fig. 1-1).

When a single-element wobbler transducer is placed in contact with the skin surface, it is rocked from side to side in a small arc by means of an electrical motor. Each individual line of the B-mode image is produced and displayed as a radius of a circle with the transducer at the center.

Beam formation in mechanical scanners is achieved through mechanical focusing using either a shaped transducer (internal focus) or an acoustic lens attached to the transducer surface (external focus) (Fig. 1-2). One of the disadvantages of this design is that the focal zone cannot be conveniently changed during scanning. Electronically focused scanners achieve focusing by delayed pulse sequences, which allow the focal zone to be changed without physically altering the scanner.

Another common design for mechanical scanners is the rotating wheel, which consists of multiple (usually two or three) transducers mounted on a wheel that is rotated by an external motor (Fig. 1-3). The wheel is rotated in the same direction, making the mechanical assembly much simpler. The wheel and transducer are housed in a fluid-filled case with an acoustic window at the lower surface that makes contact with the patient. As the transducers rotate, the output is switched from one transducer to the next in sequence, depending on which transducer has rotated in front of the acoustic window. This design allows for rapid framing without flicker—typically 30 frames per second. It produces a sector-shaped field of view and allows a wide opening angle of 90 degrees or more. It also allows the incorporation of transducers that have more than one frequency. This allows the use of lower-frequency transducers for the deeper aspects of the field of view and higher frequencies for nearer structures (Fig. 1-4).

FIGURE 1-1 Single-element mechanical sector transvaginal probes. *A.* Advanced Diagnostic Research/Advanced Technology Laboratories (ADR/ATL) transvaginal probe. *B.* Diasonics transvaginal probe. *C.* Close-up of Diasonics probe showing single-element transducer and its electrical wire.

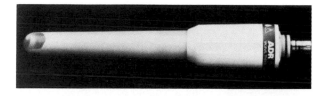

A

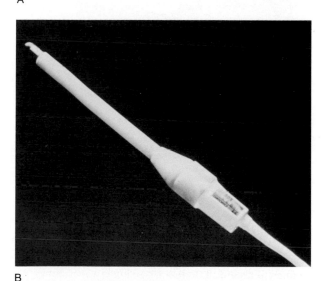

B

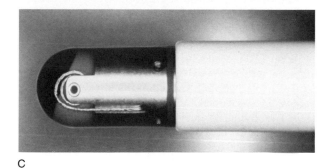

C

ELECTRONICALLY STEERED SCANNERS

Included in the category of electronically steered scanners are linear phased arrays, multi-element linear sequenced arrays, and multi-element annular arrays. Through the proper phasing of the transmit–receive timing of the transducer elements used to fabricate the arrays, a composite ultrasonic beam can be created. In this manner, the beam can be focused and steered electronically. Fundamental to electronic focusing is

FIGURE 1-2 Single-element scanners require curved transducer crystals or an attached acoustic lens to achieve focusing (top). Single-element transducers are thus focused to a specific depth (fixed focus). Array focusing is achieved by altering the times at which each subelement is pulsed, thus allowing multiple focal depths (bottom). (From Fleischer A, James AE Jr: *Diagnostic Sonography: Principles and Clinical Applications*. Philadelphia: W.B. Saunders; 1988.)

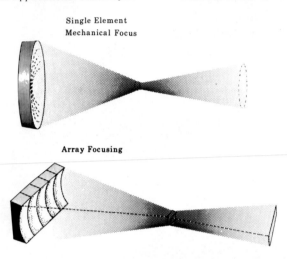

FIGURE 1-4 Rotating-wheel mechanical scanners with multiple elements provide more rapid frame rates than single-element scanners and may also produce wider fields of view. (From Fleischer A, James AE Jr: *Diagnostic Sonography: Principles and Clinical Applications*. Philadelphia: W.B. Saunders; 1988.)

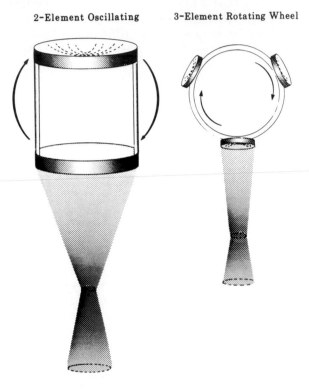

that this element of the array generates an ultrasonic wave with a definite phase relationship with the waves from the other elements. The ultrasonic waves generated by each element can be superimposed in a precise manner to create the effect of a single wavefront.

Multi-element linear sequenced arrays sequentially pulse subunits of transducers to produce a wavefront that moves normal to the transducer face, yielding a rectangular field, whereas linear phased arrays pulse all of the available transducers for each line and thus must steer as well as focus (Figs. 1-5, 1-6). An interesting and valuable variation on general field geometry is the field shape produced by curvilinear array transducers (Fig. 1-7). Radial or curvilinear arrays operate much the same as conventional linear sequenced arrays, but

FIGURE 1-3 Dual-element (5.0 and 7.5 MHz) rotating-wheel transvaginal probe (Siemens).

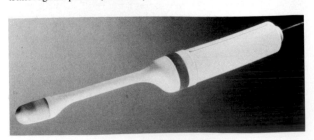

instead of being aligned in a straight line, the transducer subelements are aligned along an arc. There are several advantages to this design. By launching the ultrasound wave perpendicular to the transducer face as well as the skin, better transmission is achieved. Beam steering is achieved geometrically rather than by pulse timing, and thus eliminates the increased grating-lobe artifacts seen in phased arrays at large steering-angles, and increases the depth of the field of view, unlike conventional sequenced arrays, which produce rectangular fields of view.

The transducer array is usually composed of many (typically 128 to 256) small piezoelectric crystals (M) arranged in a row (see Fig. 1-5). Since the field from a single small crystal element diverges rapidly, several elements (N) are driven simultaneously and electronic focusing is used. In the subgroup of N crystals, the outer crystals may be pulsed first and the inner crystals delayed. Under these conditions, the field from the N elements will be focused at a depth that depends on the magnitude (time interval) of the delays. By changing the

FIGURE 1-5 Linear sequenced arrays scan the beam by sequentially pulsing transducers subgroups (N-4 illustrated) along the length of the array. Thus only a small portion of the crystals is used to form any one line. (From Fleischer A, James AE Jr: *Diagnostic Sonography: Principles and Clinical Applications*. Philadelphia: W.B. Saunders; 1988.)

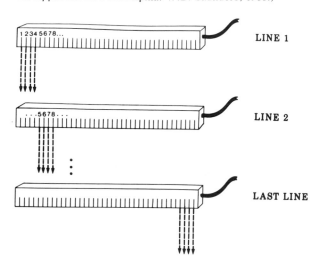

FIGURE 1-6 Linear-sequenced arrays produce rectangular fields of view and use both transmit and receive array focusing.

LINEAR PHASED ARRAY

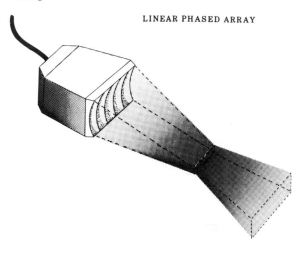

delay magnitude, the focal zone can be chosen for a specific depth. The elements may also be designed to be sensitive to the returning waves in a manner determined by the same delay factors used in transmission, thus having a focusing effect on the returning signals. A single scan line in the real-time image is formed in this manner. The next adjacent scan line is generated using another group of N crystals, formed by shifting the previous N crystals one crystal position along the transducer array. The same transmit–receive pattern is repeated for this set of N crystals, and for all other sets of N crystals along the array in a cyclic manner. Focusing in the plane of the transducer elements improves lateral resolution as well as sensitivity by increasing the amount of energy in the focal zone (constructive interference) (see Fig. 1-6). Focusing in the plane perpendicular to the scan lines determines the slice thickness and is

FIGURE 1-7 Phased curvilinear arrays are steered to produce a sector-shaped field of view and also use both transmit and receive focusing. Curvilinear arrays provide increased field of view with depth without electronic scanning, thus reducing the grating-lobe artifacts that accompany traditional phased arrays when large steering angles are used. *A.* Curvilinear array (Toshiba America Ultrasound, Inc.) transvaginal probe. The probe has needle guide attachments. *B.* The same probe with condom covering and gel coating.

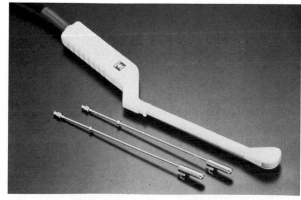

A

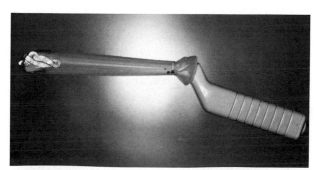

B

FIGURE 1-8   Phased-array transvaginal probe (General Electric).

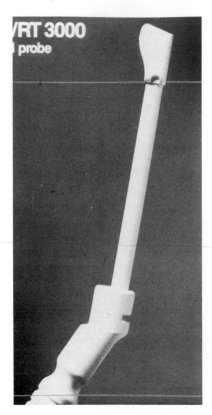

FIGURE 1-9   Diagram of side lobes produced by multi-element placed array transducers.

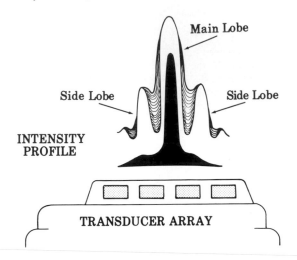

accomplished by the use of mechanically focused elements.

The linear phased array is frequently called the electronic sector scanner since the resulting field is pie-shaped with the field diverging as the distance from the transducers is increased (Figs. 1-7, 1-8). Creation of the main beam and side lobes is illustrated in Figure 1-9. The outside transducers are activated first and the inner transducers are delayed, with the central transducer delayed the most to yield a wave axis perpendicular to the plane of the transducer. By varying the order of the delay, the wave can be focused at a specified depth and the wave axis can be scanned through a sector of 60 to 90 degrees. Properly selected delays can produce steering and focusing simultaneously. One distinction between linear sequenced arrays and linear phased arrays is that in the phased array every element is used to form the beam for each line, and in the linear sequenced array only a small subset of the transducers is used to create a given line.

The phased annular array scanner is a hybrid system and has characteristics of both mechanical and electronic designs. The transducer is comprised of a series of independent transducers. Each element is shaped like an annular ring and multiple elements are arranged in concentric rings around a central transducer element (Fig. 1-10).

Beam formation and focusing is achieved electronically by proper phasing of the transducer elements. An advantage of this design is that focusing is achieved in two dimensions, similar to a single focused element, but unlike mechanical focusing, the focal zone can be changed without physically changing the transducer. Beam steering, conversely, must be achieved mechanically. The beam either is swept through a trapezoidal field of view with an oscillating mirror or the transducer may be oscillated. As with other mechanically steered scanners, the transducers, mirrors, or both are contained within a fluid-filled housing.

Commercially available annular-array scanners offer a variable focal zone option that allows the user to specify one of several focal zones. The systems also operate in a survey-scan mode in which the transducers are cyclically scanned through the available focal zones while the operator observes the images. Once a particular depth of interest is specified, the operator terminates the survey scan and selects the appropriate focal zone for optimum visualization. Scanning while the patient is on a pelvic examination table brings the structures of interest nearer to the transducer (Fig. 1-11).

Display and Storage of Real-Time Images

The number of gray shades displayed in the ultrasound image depends on the characteristics of the scan converter, which translates the pressure change received by the transducer into numbers that are stored in the

FIGURE 1-10   Phased annular arrays are capable of dynamic (both transmit [*A*] and receive [*B*] focusing and offer the added advantage that the beam is focused in two dimensions, unlike linear arrays, which are capable of electronic focusing in the plane of the array only. Receive-focus is carried out in real time by means of high-speed digital processors capable of monitoring the response received by each transducer element. By using predetermined time-delay patterns, the system can distinguish echoes that come from different depths by the relative time delays (Δt) observed by the array elements. For linear arrays, focusing in the slice-thickness direction must be accomplished mechanically. Annular arrays also must be steered mechanically. (From Fleischer A, James AE Jr: *Diagnostic Sonography: Principles and Clinical Applications*. Philadelphia: W.B. Saunders; 1988.)

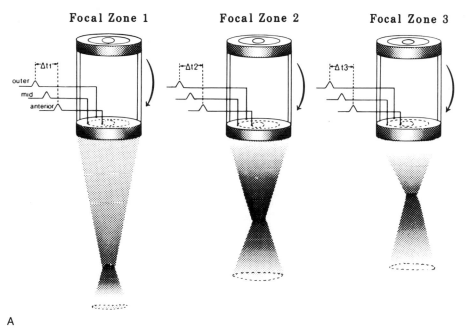

Focal Zone 1   Focal Zone 2   Focal Zone 3

A

Echo from Depth 1   Echo from Depth 2   Echo from Depth 3

B

FIGURE 1-11 A pelvic examination table is preferred but not mandatory for transvaginal sonography. Advantages of the table include support of the patient's legs and placement of the patient in a reverse Trendelenburg position, which assists collection of physiologic fluid around the uterus, tubes, and, ovaries.

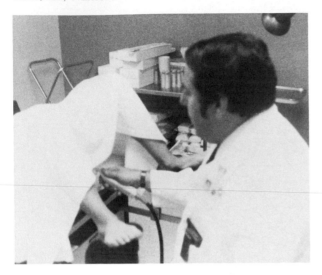

digital scan converter (Fig. 1-12). In these systems, the analog voltage levels that correspond to the returning echo amplitudes for each line of the image are digitized by an analog-to-digital converter. The generated array of numbers is then stored in a digital memory. The digital memory is divided into a number of picture elements, or pixels. The size of the memory is described by the number of pixel elements, such as 512 × 512. Each pixel represents a region in the body, the size of which is equal to the image field of view divided by the number of pixels. For example, a 25-cm field of view imaged with a 512 × 512 pixel matrix would yield pixel sizes of approximately 0.5 × 0.5 mm. The memory can then be interrogated and the image displayed on a video monitor. The brightness of the TV signal representing each picture element is controlled by the value stored in the corresponding digital word. The number of available shades of gray is determined by the size of the digital word used to store the information for each picture element. The size of the word is measured in terms of the number of bits, frequently referred to as the depth of the memory. Three-bit words provide the capacity for displaying 8 shades of gray, 4 bits provide 16 shades of gray, and 5 bits provide 32 shades of gray. Most digital memories used for real-time scanners are at least 512 × 512 by 6 to 8 bits deep (64 to 256 shades of gray).

The discreteness of both the spatial domain and the gray-scale shades provides an image that is not as smooth as the analog image. The appearance of the image will be different and the margin between picture elements pixels will be more definite than with analog displays; however, as the number of pixels increases and they become smaller, it becomes difficult to distinguish the two types of images. Images are frequently processed by linear interpolation to produce more aesthetically pleasing images. Interpolation fills in between picture elements without altering the original image data. The digital system is more stable, however, does not drift, and is less sensitive to heat, which eliminates long start-up time and allows one to institute predigital and postdigital image processing.

The most common methods for permanent archiving of ultrasound images are multiimage format film, paper print, and videotape. Multi-format film imagers have become the recording device of choice for not only ultrasound but also computed tomography, scintigraphy, and magnetic resonance imaging (Fig. 1-13A). Due to the transportability of most ultrasound systems, multi-format cameras of compact design are usually chosen. In most applications, the 9-on-1 format on 8 × 10-inch film is adequate for viewing and measurements. If larger recorded images are desired, the 6-on-1 format is also readily available. Paper printers are economical, with prints costing approximately 5 cents per print (Fig. 1-13B). They do not require processing but do not have as great a gray scale latitude as cut film.

The most recent innovation in image display involves storage of many (60 to 80) images on a single disk. These systems allow several scanners to be hooked up to a single recording device and decrease the number of trips to a processor required per day.

Videotape recorders have also become popular storage devices because they allow a real-time study to be recorded as it was performed, often with superimposed audio from the operator for further clarification of orientation and other descriptive findings.

Video recorders (VCR) using 0.5-inch VHS standard videotape are relatively inexpensive and store several hours of video on a single tape with acceptable resolution. These units generally include slow and fast motion playback modes, still-frame replay mode, and automatic search capabilities. It should be noted that in most units when still-frame imaging is used the number of displayed lines will be reduced to approximately half of the real-time display resolution. Super VHS recorders improve image resolution by increasing the number of lines in the image but are more expensive than conventional VCRs (see Fig. 1-13A).

Computerized Ultrasound

In addition to the use of digital scan converters, which has become common in current real-time systems, several manufacturers have extended the use of digital technology by replacing many of the traditional analog

FIGURE 1-12 Block diagram of a digital ultrasound system. Echo signals detected by the transducer are digitized and then stored in a computer memory (digital scan converter), which is read out to a video monitor. (From Fleischer A, James AE Jr: *Diagnostic Sonography: Principles and Clinical Applications*. Philadelphia: W.B. Saunders; 1988.)

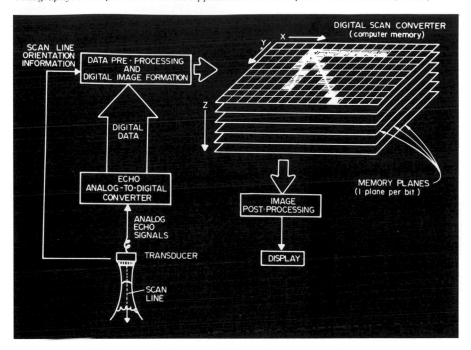

portions of the system's pulsing and receiving hardware. In the past it has been appreciated that digital components provide flexibility through software programmability that analog systems cannot. Only recently have the price and speed of digital systems been such that the replacement of analog circuits could be considered, however. High-speed parallel processors under program-control driving multi-element array transducers have made it possible to dynamically vary pulsing and receiving signal processing steps. This differs from analog circuits, which must be physically changed each time a change in signal processing is made.

As described previously, a beam can be formed and steered by pulse timing of transducer arrays. The beam will have a focal depth that depends on the values of the time delays between the pulsing of the outer transducer elements relative to the center elements. Once a beam is launched from the transducer it cannot be controlled further. In the case of transmit focus the primary benefit of digital flexibility benefit is that it allows one to choose the focal zone before each scan without having to physically change the transducers. This is an important practical benefit but does not change the resultant image quality compared with analog systems.

The most significant improvement in image quality

that has resulted directly from the use of digital systems has been the benefit derived from dynamic signal processing on the returning echoes. This is often referred to as receive focusing or dynamic focusing. Although the transmitted beam can have only a single focal zone, it is possible to selectively "listen" to the returning echoes. Returning echoes from different depths arrive at different times, that is, nearby reflections are detected first, followed by reflection from deeper sites. Accepting only those echoes that have the proper pattern of arrival times ensures that the returning signals are in focus for each depth. This is the essence of dynamic focusing. To accomplish dynamic focusing, it is essential that the system have almost complete control over the pulsing and receiving of each individual transducer element, which requires the power of high speed parallel processing. Conventional multi-element scanners sum the received signal with equal weightings from the various elements to produce the echo signal. In the parallel processed systems, the gain of each element is controlled separately. This dynamically variable gain capability is referred to as dynamic apodization. Dynamic variations in the individual gains can be used to discard echoes from off-axis sites to minimize side lobe and grating lobe artifacts. The same technique can also be used to effectively change the size of the aperture during the

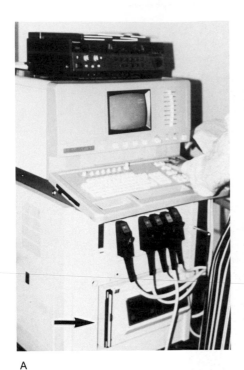

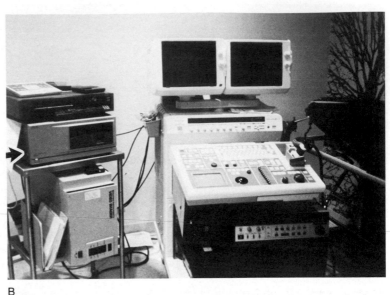

FIGURE 1-13   Recording devices. *A.* Multiformat camera (arrow) for recording hard-copy film. A VCR is used for videotaping on top of Acuson 280. *B.* Paper printer for color and black-and-white paper prints attached to Toshiba 270 scanner (arrow).

A   B

scan depending on whether one is scanning in the near or far field.

Endoluminal Transducer-Probes

Recent advances in transducer designs have resulted in development of transducers that can be mounted on probes and placed within various lumen of the body. The two major types of endoluminal probes that have gained clinical application include transvaginal transducer-probes for imaging of the uterus, early pregnancy, and the adnexa; and transrectal transducer-probes for imaging of the cervix, uterus, and parametrium.

Because of the proximity of the organ of interest to the transducer, both transvaginal and transrectal probes can use transducers with frequencies of 5 or 7.5 MHz. In general, the use of these probes can contribute to increased diagnostic specificity by the improved resolution afforded by the proximity of the transducer to the area of interest and the higher transducer frequencies that can be used.

Transvaginal transducer-probes significantly enhance the sonographic evaluation of the uterus and adnexa. There are between 10 and 15 different types of commercially available probes (Table 1-1) (Platt, 1987). The major types of transvaginal probes include those that use a single-element mechanical oscillating trans-

ducer, those with a curved linear array, those that use an electronically phased steering of multiple transducer elements, and those that use a single-element transducer that rotates (see Figs. 1-1 to 1-9).

In general, the field of view of most transvaginal probes is approximately 10 cm, with the focal range varying from 2 to 7 cm depending on the type and design of the transducers. The sector of the field of view is typically 90 to 100 degrees, with some rotating wheel designs going as high as 240 degrees. The design of the actual probe housing ranges from a straight shaft with a transducer mounted on the end to ones in which the transducer's face is inclined relative to the handle.

Needle guides are available on several transvaginal transducer-probes that attach to the shaft (Fig. 1-14). Some are flush with the shape of the probe, whereas others are outrigged (see Fig. 1-14*A* to *D*). When probes with an outrigged needle guide are used care must be taken not to press on the area of the anterior urethra. The path of the needle can be superimposed on the imaging monitor, thereby providing precise guidance for a variety of interventional procedures such as a follicular or cyst aspiration.

When determining which transvaginal transducer-probe to use, one should remember that each varies according to the size of the actual contact surface or footprint, the size of the shaft, and the angle of the handle. Handles that assist the operator in determining

Table 1-1   High-Level Disinfectant Products

Manufacturer	Brand Name	Effect on Microorganisms
Sporicidin International 12000 Old Georgetown Road Rockville, MD 20852	Sporicidin disinfectant spray* Sporicidin disinfectant solution* Sporicidin towelettes*	Herpes 1 and 2, polio 1 and 2, Coxsackie virus B-1 cytomegalovirus, Rotavirus, HIV-1, influenza A2 parvovirus, vaccinia, *Bacillus subtilis, Clostridum sporogenes*
Central Solutions, Inc. 3130 Brinkerhoff Road Box 15276 Kansas City, KS 66115	Pheno-Cen disinfectant spray*	*Salmonella choleraesuis, Trichophyton mentagrophytes, Staphylococcus aureus, Pseudomonas aeruginosa* HIV-1
Surgikos, Inc. P.O. Box 130 Arlington, TX 76010	Cidex Plus disinfectant solution* Cidex disinfectant solution*	Herpes 1 and 2, HIV-1, cytomegalovirus, adenovirus type 2, poliovirus type 1, rhinovirus, coxsackievirus B1, *B. subtilis, C. sporogenes*
Metrex Research Corporation 11270 South Dranfeldt Road P.O. Box 965 Parker, CO 80134	MetriCide 28 disinfectant solution* MetriCide disinfectant solution*	Herpes 1 and 2, HIV-1, cytomegalovirus, rhinovirus vaccinia, adenovirus, *T. mentagrophytes, Mycobacterium bovis, S. aureus, S. Choleraesuis*

*Registered with the EPA as an inactivator of HIV-1.
From Odwin C, Fleischer A, Kepple D, et al. Probe covers and disinfectants for transvaginal transducers. *JDMS* 1990;6:130–135.

probe orientation are preferred. Probes with the smallest shaft size may be preferred in virgins or young girls and older women with less distensible vaginas.

Transrectal probes are used extensively for prostate evaluation (Fig. 1-15A), but can be used for guidance of circlage, intrauterine tandem placement, guided dilation and curretage, or intrauterine contraceptive device retrieval (Fleischer et al, 1990). These probes usually contain at least one array of transducers. For imaging in the sagittal plane, a series of linear array elements with electronic or phased-array focusing is usually used. For those probes that have two elements, the axial view is usually obtained by a single-element mechanically oscillated transducer, curved linear array, or phased-array transducer array (Fig. 1-15B).

Transducers that can be placed on an examiner's fingertip are now being developed (Fig. 1-16). These also may have biplanar imaging capabilities with a curvilinear array mounted at the top of the housing and a slightly curved linear array below.

Doppler Systems

Doppler systems have evolved from the relatively simple continuous wave (CW) units, which yielded an audible frequency to the users' earphones, to current pulsed-Doppler systems capable of yielding color-coded flow images in real time. This evolution has been made possible in large part by the advent of relatively inexpensive high-speed parallel-processing computers. The basic interaction of the Doppler effect has not changed over the years, but our ability to rapidly process and analyze the returning echo data has improved (Taylor, 1987).

Ultrasound passing through the body is either absorbed (a decrease in beam intensity of about 1 dB/cm/MHz) or reflected. Ultrasound is reflected at each point along the beam where the relative acoustical impedance changes. If this reflecting interface is stationary, the frequency of the reflected wave will be identical to the incident beam. If the interface is moving, the reflected echo frequency will be shifted up or down (relative to the incident wave) by an amount proportional to the velocity along the beam direction. This shift is called the Doppler shift and is given by the following equation:

$$\Delta f = \frac{\pm 2Vf_0}{c} \cos \theta$$

where Δf = Doppler shift frequency (Hz)
V = velocity of the moving interface (cm/sec)
f_0 = frequency of the incident sound (Hz)
c = velocity of sound in tissue (cm/sec)
θ = the angle in degrees between the sound beam direction and the direction of the moving interface

Their actual received frequency (*fr*) from the moving interface is:

$$fr = f_0 \pm \Delta f$$

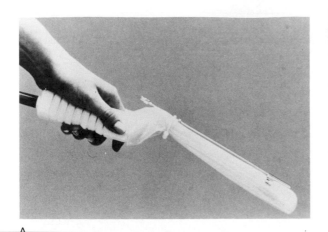

A

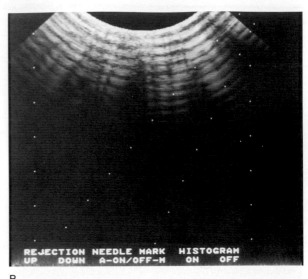

B

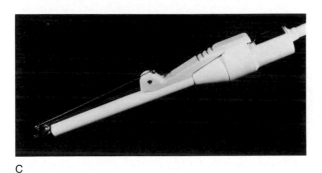

C

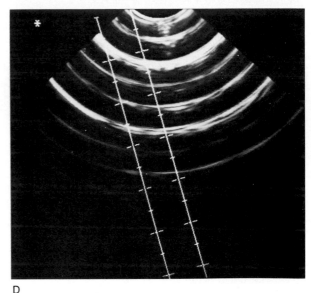

D

FIGURE 1-14   Needle guides. *A*. Needle-guide attachment to a curvilinear array transvaginal probe. *B*. Needle path display on imaging monitor. *C*. Mechanical sector transvaginal probe with "outrigged" needle guide. *D*. Needle path display on imaging monitor.

When the impinging ultrasound beam passes through a blood vessel, scattering of the ultrasound wave occurs. In this process, small amounts of sound energy are absorbed by each red cell and reradiated in all directions. If the red blood cell is moving with respect to the source, the backscattered energy returning to the receiving transducer will be shifted in frequency; the magnitude and direction of this shift is proportional to the velocity of the respective cell. If the ultrasound beam is considered to fill the entire lumen of a blood vessel, then the backscattered signal will consist of all the Doppler shifts produced by the red cells moving through the ultrasonic beam. Since there is always a range of velocities present, from zero at the vessel wall to a peak value near the center of the vessel lumen, a spectrum of Doppler shift frequencies is always present. The frequency spectrum is derived by applying a mathematical operation, called a Fourier transformation, to the returning echo wave train. This spectrum can become complex with pulsating blood flow and vessel wall motion, especially when blood flow disturbances due to anatomic defects are present. Vessel wall irregularity, ulcerated plaques, narrowed or partially occluded vessels, or other abnormalities such as stenotic heart valves cause velocity variation that can be readily detected by differences in the frequency spectrum of the Doppler signal.

FIGURE 1-15   A biplane transrectal probe. *A*. This transrectal probe with biplanar capability has both linear and sector scanners incorporated into a single probe. *B*. Diagram of field of view and scan-plane orientations for the dual transducer transrectal probe.

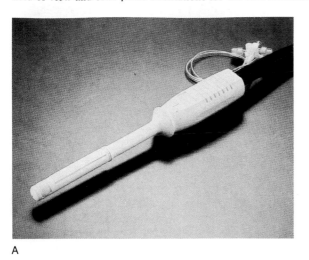

A

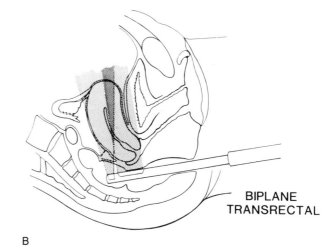

BIPLANE
TRANSRECTAL

B

A number of imaging schemes have been devised to give the user some information on the vessel anatomy in addition to blood flow. The simplest of these uses a CW Doppler transducer fixed to a mechanical arm. As the transducer moves over a vessel of interest, an image corresponding to each site of inquiry is produced on a storage oscilloscope. A serious deficiency of this simple continuous wave (CW) Doppler instrument is of depth resolution.

The most practical means to add depth resolution to a Doppler instrument is to pulse the source and add a range gate to the receiver. These pulsed Doppler devices are similar to a pulse-echo instrument in that bursts of ultrasound are emitted at a regular rate into the body tissue. A new pulse will not be transmitted until echoes from the previous pulse have ceased or significantly diminished. The depth of a pulse can be determined by noting the time of its flight to an interface and its return. Relatively short bursts of approximately 0.5 to 1.0 μsec can be used to give high axial resolution for detection of the location and separation of interfaces to within 1 mm or less.

The principle of pulsed Doppler is different from that of a pulse-echo instrument. To determine the

FIGURE 1-16   Finger-tip transducers. *A*. Finger-"top" curvilinear array transducer. *B*. Longitudinally oriented curved linear array. (Courtesy of Hitachi Corporation.)

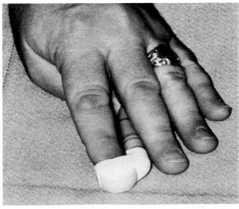

A

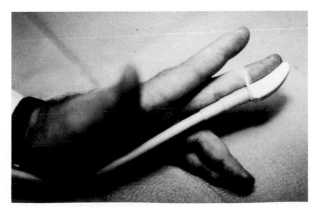

B

Doppler spectrum of a reflected wave from many depths simultaneously in real time requires extremely fast parallel processes needed to carry out the many calculations needed to arrive at the frequency shift of each pixel. Because of the relatively long time needed to perform a Fourier transformation, faster phase sensitive calculations are often used instead. To display these multi-dimensional data (flow magnitude, direction, and location) color-coded images are often used. In the image, color is used to encode direction and hue is used to encode relative magnitude. Red colors are usually assigned to flow toward the transducer; blue is used for flow away from the transducer, and whiter colors represent high frequency shifts in areas of flow with increased velocities. Turbulent flow can be imaged as a mosaic pattern displayed in shades of yellow and green.

A disadvantage of pulsed Doppler scanners is their inability to accurately determine rapid flow. Consequently they may present alaised results in which a high-flow location is actually presented as a low-flow location. The maximum flow measured by a pulsed Doppler system is determined by the pulse repetition (PRF) of the system. Specifically, the detected Doppler shift frequency (Δf) can not be greater than PRF/2. Increasing PRF to allow estimates of rapid flow limits the field of view to superficial structures and also adds the potential for range ambiguity errors. Range ambiguity errors occur when echoes from previous lines are received as echoes from the current line (Gill et al, 1989). Fortunately flow aliasing can often be recognized and generally will not lead to mistaken diagnoses.

Quality Control

The purpose of a quality assurance program is to ensure that the diagnostic quality of all ultrasonic images is maintained at the maximum attainable level. Part of this program must include monitoring procedures that ensure the proper and consistent operation of all equipment. Equipment acceptance tests must be performed on new equipment and repeated whenever major equipment repairs are made. Quality assurance tests should be performed on a routine basis to detect deviations from the baseline acceptance tests. Quality assurance is the joint responsibility of the sonologist, sonographer, and service support personnel.

There are numerous test objects and instruments available for assessing the performance of ultrasonic equipment. A number of documents are also available that contain detailed protocols for establishing a quality assurance program. Probably the single most versatile and complete test object is the American Institute of Ultrasound in Medicine (AIUM) Standard 100 mm Test Object. The standard AIUM Test Object is filled with a relatively nonattenuating medium. Phantoms with a similar configuration but filled with an attenuating tissue-equivalent material are also commercially available. These tissue-equivalent phantoms provide system beam-parameter measurements in a more clinically pertinent situation (Fig. 1-17A,B). The ability to discern closely spaced wires in the far field corresponds to axial resolution capabilities, whereas the width of the echo returned from centrally placed wires corresponds to lateral resolution properties. The ability to depict variously sized cysts as shown within the soft tissue matrix correlates to the ability to discern cystic structures within organs.

A minimal quality assurance program should include routine monitoring of the performance of the gray scale photography, the image system sensitivity, the axial resolution, and the accuracy and linearity of distance markers. In addition to evaluation of the gray scale system, the AIUM Test Object may be used to assess each of the other system parameters. The minimal quality assurance program provides relative parameter values, which are useful for detecting early changes in image system characteristics. Absolute measurements of system parameters are more difficult and may require additional test objects and equipment.

Of equal importance to the actual performance testing is documentation of the test results. These recorded data are essential for accurate monitoring of equipment performance, and are useful to both the equipment service personnel and the equipment manufacturer. It is also possible that this will be required by government regulatory and certifying agencies in the near future.

The initial camera settings, scan converter output controls, or both largely depend on individual points of reference. Once a baseline has been established, a daily evaluation should be made to ensure that the same range of echo amplitudes as previous test exposures can be seen.

Most systems now generate a gray scale bar displayed to one side or at the bottom of the image. This bar should be examined daily for consistency of step distribution and display. The comparison can be made either by visual inspection or with the aid of a densitometer, which is more quantitative.

A simple test for system sensitivity stability can be performed with the AIUM phantom. After carefully positioning the transducer directly above the reference wires, which are spaced 2 cm apart, and, after making sure the transducer face is flat against the phantom surface, the system gain (attenuation or output) settings should be adjusted to display a one-division echo from the most distant wire. The gain setting should not change on subsequent recordings. Similarly, the minimum gain

FIGURE 1-17   Phantom. *A*. Photograph of soft tissue-cyst phantom. *B*. Image from phantom illustrating axial resolution as ability to depict closely spaced wires (short arrow), lateral resolution of beam as size of the center dot (long arrow), and cysts within soft tissue matrix. (Courtesy of Nuclear Associates.)

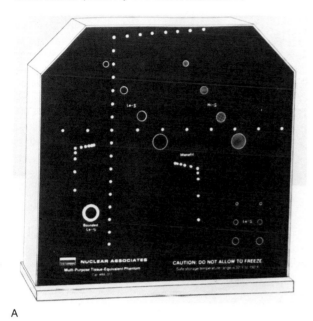

A

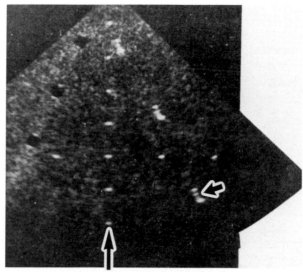

B

settings required to yield a discernible echo in the B-mode image should not change with time. This method determines the stability of the instrumentation over time.

A single image of the AIUM phantom provides data on axial resolution as well as the accuracy and linearity of the distance markers. Axial resolution is assessed from the minimum resolvable spacing in the set of diagonal wires at the center of the phantom. Within this set, wire spacings range from 5 mm to 1 mm. Most imaging systems should exhibit the ability to resolve 2-mm wire spacings and this value should remain constant over time.

The accuracy and linearity of the system-generated distance markers can be evaluated by a direct measurement of the distances of the vertical and horizontal wires from a B-mode image. The distance between the top and bottom wires in the 2-cm spaced groups is actually 10 cm, and this distance, as estimated by the markers, should not differ by more than 2 mm.

Bioeffects Considerations

Theoretical extrapolation from bioeffects that have occurred at intensities and magnitudes higher than that used for diagnostic sonography has suggested a threshold

for possible production of bioeffects at 100 mW/cm^2. There has never been a biologically significant adverse bioeffect attributed to diagnostic ultrasound, however (Merritt, 1989).

Manufacturers must report the intensities used for diagnostic imaging, duplex, and color Doppler imaging. Most manufacturers have complied with the Food and Drug Administration recommendation of intensities lower than 94 mW/cm^2. Before purchasing a transvaginal probe one should ask the manufacturer for data concerning the intensities used.

Some believe that transvaginal sonography with the probe nearer to the embryo than in conventional sonographic scanning delivers more of the incident beam to potentially sensitive tissue. Since higher frequencies and more well-focused beams are used for transvaginal sonography, however, less of the incident beam is actually propagated (Goldstein, 1989).

One may postulate that excessive pressure on a follicle-bearing ovary or hemorrhagic ovarian mass could potentiate rupture or torsion. No reports of this have been published. A more likely complication, however, is the potential for infection when the probe is not properly prepared with a bacteriostatic medium between studies. We recommend the use of a bacteriostatic spray (Sporocidin) applied to the probe after each study

Table 1-2   Manufacturers' Recommendations* for Disinfection or Sterilization of Transvaginal Transducers

Manufacturer	Recommendations	Precautionary Measures
Acuson	Cidex, MetriCide, Microbac, Sporicidin	Do not ultraviolet sterilize. Do not gas or dry heat sterilize. Do not autoclave. Do not use chlorine bleach. Do not use iodine compounds to clean or wipe.
Ausonics	Sporicidin	When using diluted bleach do not immerse. Wipe quickly and use water to clean any residue.
Diasonics	Cidex, Sporicidin, or chlorine bleach	Use bleach only in an emergency situation as bleach could damage the steel jacket.
ATL	Cidex or Sporicidin	Immerse transducer tip only, do not immerse handle. Do not gas or heat sterilize. Do not allow solution to enter strain relief joint or tracking adjustment slot.
Siemens	Chlorhexidinegluconat (Hibitance) Cidex, Gigasept	Follow the manufacturers' directions. Never use phenol or other organic-based solvent. Never use heat-steam or cold gas (ethylene oxide).
Toshiba	Formalin or ethylene oxide gas, chlorhexidine (Hibitance) 0.5%, hypochlorous sodium 0.1%, glutaraldehyde 2% (Cidex), Sporicidin	Diluted bleach (1 part bleach per 10 parts water). After disinfecting, rinse with sterile water.

*Use of any of the following products against manufacturer instructions or precautionary measures could void the transducer warranty.
From Odwin C, Fleischer A, Kepple D, et al. Probe covers and disinfectants for transvaginal transducers. *JDMS* 1990;6:130–135.

Table 1-3   Disposable Probe Covers for Transvaginal Transducers

Manufacturer	Brand	Talc	Precautions
CIVCO Medical Instruments, Inc. 418 B Avenue, Drawer Q Kalona, IA 52247	Latex*	Yes†	Can be damaged by heat or light; store in dark, cool, dry place. Do not lubricate with petroleum-based lubricants.
	Polyethylene*	No	
	CIV-Flex (polyurethane)*	No	Nonembryotoxic
	Enviro-Flex (polyethylene)*	No	
Schmid Laboratories, Inc. Little Falls, NJ 07424	Latex condom (Ramses)	Yes†	Avoid prolonged storage at temperatures above 100°F; do not lubricate with oil-based lubricants; can be damaged by heat or light.
Carter-Wallace, Inc. New York, NY 10153	Latex condom (Trojans)	Yes†	Avoid prolonged storage at temperatures above 100°F; do not lubricate with oil-based lubricants; can be damaged by heat or light.

*Approved by the FDA for transducers.
†Minimal amount.
From Odwin C, Fleischer A, Kepple D, et al. Probe covers and disinfectants for transvaginal transducers. *JDMS* 1990;6:130–135.

(Odwin, 1990); however, each manufacturer has specific recommendations for disinfection of their transducers.

Probe Preparation, Covers, and Gel

There are several products and methods for disinfection of transvaginal and transrectal probes (see Table 1-1). The most practical and efficacious one involves spraying the probe with a disinfectant before use. Sporocidin is sufficiently bacteriostatic and virostatic (including the human immunodeficiency [HIV] virus) since it kills on contact (Odwin et al, 1990). The use of this spray does not require that the probe sit in disinfectant. Since each probe is made to different specifications, each manufacturer recommends a specific method for disinfection (Table 1-2).

Latex condoms can be used as probe covers (Table 1-3). To secure the condom with sufficient tension to the probe, it can be twisted over the shaft before it is secured with rubber bands.

There are a variety of acoustic gels used for transvaginal scanning. A sufficient amount of gel needs to be placed both within and around the condom to provide adequate acoustic coupling. Some gels may affect sperm motility and should not be used in patients undergoing insemination. The reader is referred to the review article by Odwin et al for more information.

Summary

This chapter has discussed and illustrated the pivotal and clinically pertinent principles involved in transvaginal and transrectal sonographic imaging. An understanding of the probe design can optimize transvaginal imaging with these transducer probes.

References

Fleischer A, Burnett L, Jones H. Guidance for intraoperative uterine procedures with transrectal sonography. *Radiology* 1990;176:576–577.

Gill RW, Kossoff MB, Kossoff G, Griffiths KA. New class of pulsed Doppler US ambiguity at short ranges. *Radiology* 1989;173:272–275.

Goldstein A. Advances in transducer technology, digital circuitry and software have enhanced ultrasound image quality. *Diagn Imaging* 1989;11.

Merritt C. Ultrasound safety: what are the issues? *Radiology* 1989;173:304.

Odwin C, Fleischer A, Kepple D, et al. Probe covers and disinfectants for transvaginal transducers. *J Diagn Med Sonog* 1990;6:130–135.

Platt LD. New look in ultrasound: the vaginal probe. *Contemp Obstet Gynecol* October 1987;30:99–105.

Taylor KJW. Going to the depths with duplex Doppler. *Diagn Imaging* October 1987;9:106.

Chapter 2

Normal Pelvic Anatomy and Scanning Techniques

Arthur C. Fleischer, MD
Donna M. Kepple, RDMS

Introduction

Transvaginal sonography (TVS) affords better resolution of the uterus and ovaries than that obtained with the conventional transabdominal approach (TAS). Although the proximity of the transducer-probe to the pelvic organs allows detailed depiction, it may be more (rather than less) difficult for the sonographer to become oriented to the images obtained on a transvaginal sonogram compared with conventional TAS. This is because of the limited field of view and unusual scanning planes depicted with TVS (Fig. 2-1A,B).

As a systematic approach for examining the uterus and adnexal structures develops, the examination becomes much easier to perform. Our usual protocol begins with depiction of the uterus in long axis in a sagittal plane, followed by delineation of the adnexae in a semicoronal or semiaxial plane. The last images are obtained of the cervix and cul-de-sac as the transducer is withdrawn from the vaginal fornices.

In this chapter, the sonographic appearances of the uterus, ovary, and other adnexal and pelvic structures will be described with particular emphasis on how they are best depicted on a real-time TVS examination.

Scanning Technique and Instrumentation

The three scanning maneuvers used in TVS include:

1. Vaginal insertion of the probe with side-to-side movement within the upper vagina for oblique saggital imaging (Fig. 2-2A).
2. Transverse orientation of the probe for imaging of the adnexa and uterus in various degrees of semiaxial to semicoronal planes (Fig. 2-2B). In most patients the adnexa is best examined in this plane.
3. Variation in depth of probe insertion for optimal imaging of the fundus and corpus. Imaging of the cervix is optimized by gradual withdrawal of the probe into the midvagina (Fig. 2-2C).

Other maneuvers, such as placing the patient in a decubitus position to bring a floating yolk sac/embryo closer to the probe, can be used in selected cases.

As opposed to conventional TAS, bladder distension is not required for TVS. In fact, over-distension can hinder TVS by placing the desired field of view outside of the optimal focal range of the transducer. Minimal distension is useful in patients with severely anteflexed uteri; it straightens them out relative to the imaging plane.

As with conventional sonographic equipment, one should select the highest frequency transducer possible that allows adequate penetration and depiction of a particular region of interest. Thus, 5.0 and 7.5 MHz transducers are preferred, but these higher frequency transducers limit the field of view to within 6 to 8 cm of the probe.

The major types of transducer-probes used for transvaginal scanning include those that contain a single-element oscillating transducer, those with multiple small transducer elements arranged in a curved linear array, and those that consist of multiple small elements steered by an electronically phased array (see Chapter 1). All of these depict the anatomy in a sector format encompassing between 85 and 100 degrees. In our experience, the greatest resolution is achieved with a curved linear array that contains multiple (up to 124) separate transmit–receive elements. Mechanical sector transducers may be subject to minor image distortions at the edges of the field due to the hysteresis (stopping and starting)

FIGURE 2-1 Comparison of transabdominal and transvaginal pelvic sonography with diagrams and images. *A.* Sector seen in TVS superimposed on a transabdominal pelvic sonogram. *B.* Transvaginal image showing field of view depicted in *A.*

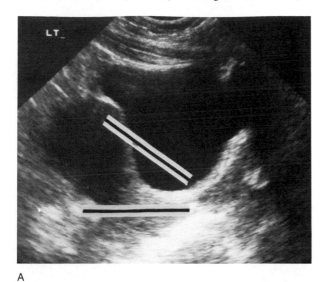

A

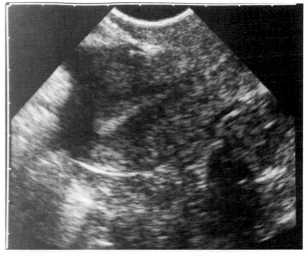

B

FIGURE 2-2 Scanning planes used in TVS. *A.* Oblique sagittal planes. *B.* Semicoronal planes. *C.* Diagrams showing field of view with various degrees of probe insertion. Varying the degree of probe penetration alters the field of view. (Courtesy of Bill Carrano.)

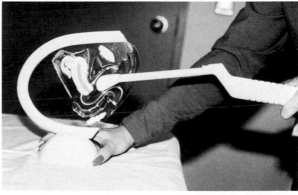

A

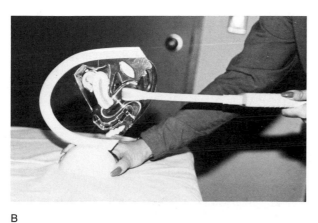

B

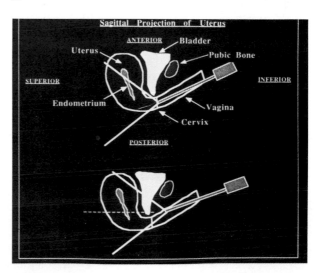

C

FIGURE 2-3   Artifacts. *A.* Reverberation artifact (curved arrow) projected over bladder. *B.* Same artifact displayed as if within gestational sac.

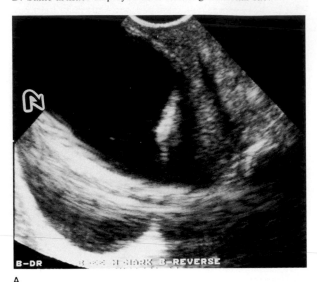

A

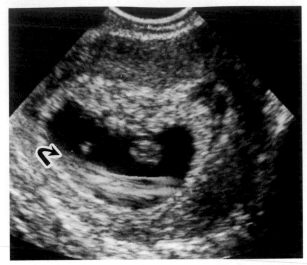

B

that occurs with an oscillating transducer. Reverberation artifacts can be created by suboptimal coupling of the condom/probe/vagina surfaces (Fig. 2-3*A,B*) or lack of tautness of the condom as it is stretched over the probe. Although degradation of image quality by side lobe artifacts can occur in the far field in a phased-array transducer, the image in the near field is not degraded significantly. Therefore, phased array transducers have resolution capabilities similar to sector and curved linear transducers when used in transvaginal examinations.

After complete covering of the transducer probe by a condom and securement of the condom to the shaft of the probe by a rubber band, the probe is inserted within the vagina and manipulated around the cervical lips and into a fornix to depict the structures of interest in the most detail. When the transducer is oriented in the longitudinal or sagittal plane, the long axis of the uterus can usually be depicted by slight oblique angulation off midline. The uterus is used as a landmark for depiction of other adnexal structures. Once the uterus is identified, the probe can be angled to the right or left of midline in the sagittal plane to depict the ovaries. The internal iliac artery and vein appear as tubular structures along the pelvic sidewall. Low-level blood echoes can occasionally be seen streaming within these pulsating vessels. The ovaries typically lie medial to these vessels. Hypoechoic follicles within the ovaries facilitate their identification. After appropriate images are obtained in the sagittal plane, the transducer can be turned 90 degrees counterclockwise to depict these

structures in their axial or semicoronal planes. Counterclockwise movement maintains standard right-to-left orientation on the semicoronal scans.

Particularly in larger patients, it is helpful for the sonographer to use one hand to scan while the other is used for gentle abdominal palpation so as to move structures such as the ovaries as close as possible to the transducer and also to displace bowel.

Occasionally placement of the patient in a decubitus position is helpful in bringing the area of interest closer to the transducer. This maneuver is particularly used in early pregnancy when the yolk sac/embryo complex may lie in the far field or on the edge of the sac. Left-lateral decubitus positioning is easier than right for the patient and examiner.

A pelvic examination table is preferred for TVS primarily because the legs are supported, thus enabling the patient to relax her abdominal, leg, and perineal muscles (Fig. 2-4). If one is not available, an inverted bed pan can be placed under the patient's buttocks to elevate the pelvis from the stretcher surface. This allows the examiner to displace the handle posteriorly to direct the probe and beam anteriorly.

Scanning Planes

TVS affords examination of the pelvic organs in three major imaging planes: sagittal, semicoronal, and semiaxial. The sagittal plane is usually used initially to

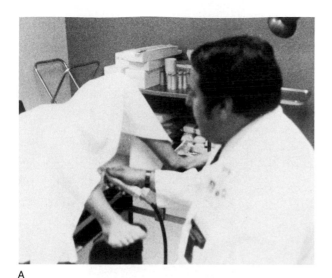

A

FIGURE 2-4   Equipment used for TVS. *A.* Patient on pelvic examination table in slight reverse Trendelenburg position. This position affords collection of physiologic fluid in the cul-de-sac and allows the patient's legs to be supported. *B.* Transvaginal transducer-probe covered with a condom. A small amount of gel is placed on the condom to facilitate insertion and contact.

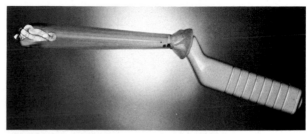

B

identify the uterus in the long axis. Once this structure is adequately depicted, the transducer probe can be directed into the right or left adnexa, where the ovary and iliac vessels are seen. One can use various degrees of pressure on the probe to move the organs of interest closest to the transducer while displacing bowel. The semicoronal and semiaxial images are then obtained by turning the probe 90 degrees counterclockwise. If the probe is directed in the coronal plane, it is termed a semicoronal image. Semiaxial images are obtained when the beam is directed anteriorly. Finally, a posteriorly directed image of the cul-de-sac is obtained when the probe is withdrawn from the vaginal fornices into the mid-vagina. The reader is encouraged to refer to the line drawings to get a better appreciation of these scanning planes.

Image Display

To distinguish a transvaginal sonogram from a conventional transabdominal one, "TV" should be displayed at the top left of the screen. For oblique sagittal and semicoronal images, the main bang should be displayed at the top of the screen with the cephalic direction displayed to the left of the screen. For semicoronal planes, the patient's right should be displayed on the left of the screen. Admittedly, neither display from the top or the bottom of the screen is anatomically correct, but this method of display fits closest to that already established as convention by the American Institute of Ultrasound in Medicine and has been used extensively in this country.

Uterus

Examination of the uterus begins with its depiction in long axis. The endometrial interface, which is typically echogenic, is a useful landmark to depict the long axis of the uterus. Once the endometrium is identified, images of the uterus can be obtained in the sagittal and semiaxial/ coronal plane. In the oblique sagittal plane, an anteflexed uterus will display the fundus to the left of the image; the reverse is true for a retroflexed uterus (Fig. 2-5).

It may be difficult to determine the flexion of the uterus on the hard-copy images obtained from transvaginal scanning alone, except in extreme cases of ante- or retroflexion. One can obtain an impression of a uterine flexion during the examination, however, by the relative orientation of the transducer probe needed to obtain the most optimal images of the uterus. For example, retroflexed uteri are best depicted when the probe is in the anterior fornix and angulated in a posterior direction.

The endometrium has a variety of appearances depending on its stage of development (Fleischer, 1988). In the proliferative phase, the endometrium measures 4 to 8 mm in anteroposterior (AP) dimension (width). This measurement includes two layers of endometrium. A hypoechoic interface can be seen within the luminal aspects of echogenic layers of endometrium in the periovulatory phase and probably represents an edema in the inner layers of endometrium. In the few days after ovulation, a small amount of secretion into the endometrial lumen can be seen. During the secretory phase, the endometrium typically measures 8 to 14 mm in width and is surrounded by a hypoechoic band

FIGURE 2-5   Uterus

2-5A   Long axis of uterus and endometrium (between cursors) in secretory phase appearing as echogenic tissue. A nabothian cyst is also present.

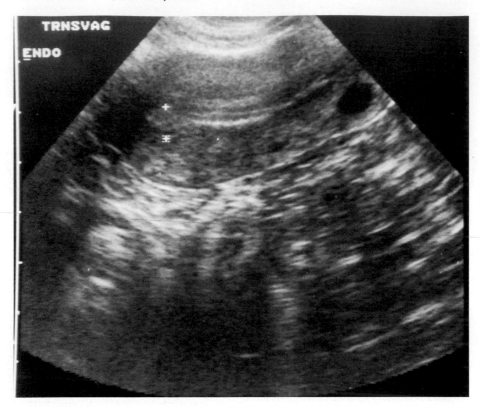

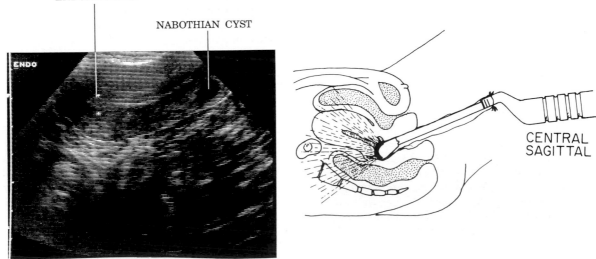

ENDOMETRIUM

NABOTHIAN CYST

CENTRAL
SAGITTAL

FIGURE 2-5   Uterus *(continued)*

2-5B   Same as *A* in semicoronal short axis.

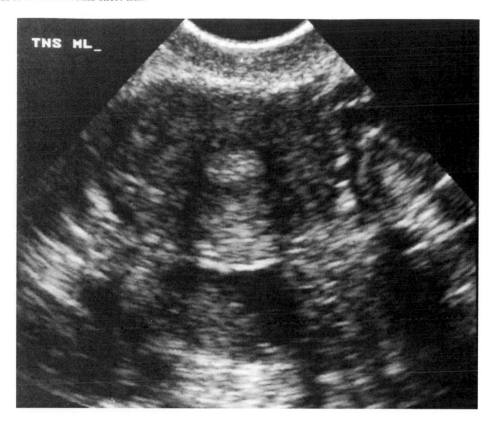

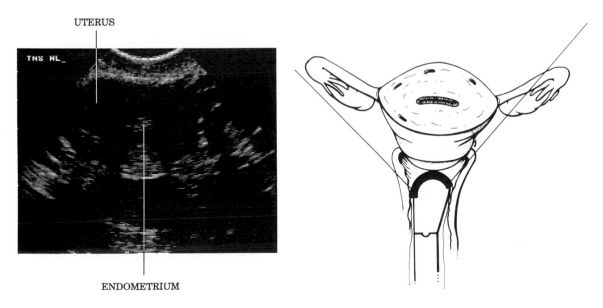

UTERUS

ENDOMETRIUM

(continued)

FIGURE 2-5   Uterus *(continued)*

2-5C   Saggital image showing penetrating vessels within the outer myometrium at level of internal cervical os.

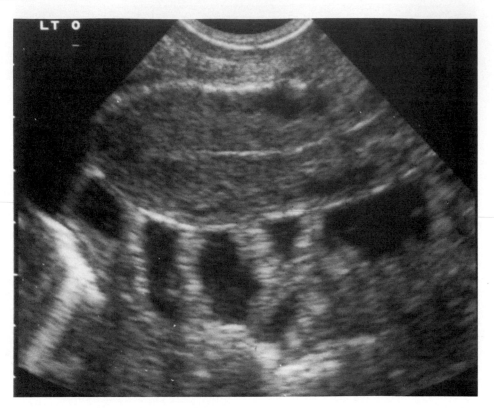

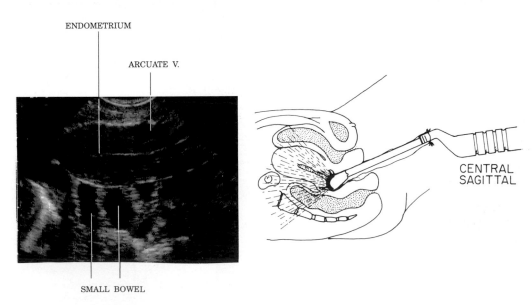

representing the inner layer of the myometrium. One is reminded to measure the endometrium only in a straight sagittal image; measuring it in a semicoronal image is inaccurate.

An endometrial volume may be calculated by measuring its length by long axis, with AP and transverse dimensions. One can use the landmark in the axial plane where the endometrium invaginates into the area of ostia in the region of the uterine cornu.

Because of the proximity of the transducer probe to the cervix, the cervix is not as readily depicted as the remainder of the uterus. If one withdraws the probe into the vagina while maintaining visualization of the endometrium, however, images of the cervix can be obtained. The mucus within the endocervical canal usually appears as an echogenic interface. This may become hypoechoic during the periovulatory period, because the cervical mucus has a higher fluid content.

Ovaries

Ovaries are typically depicted as oblong structures measuring approximately 3 cm in long-axis and 2 cm in AP and transverse dimension (Fig. 2-6). On angled long-axis scans, they are immediately medial to the pelvic vessels. They are particularly well depicted when they contain a mature follicle that is typically in the 1.5 to 2.0 cm range. It is not unusual to depict multiple immature or atretic follicles in the 3 to 5 mm range that serve as sonographic markers of the ovary.

The size of an ovary is related to the patient's age and phase of follicular development (Granberg, 1987). When the ovary contains a mature follicle, it can become twice as large in volume as one that does not contain mature follicles. The ovaries of postmenopausal women are usually small (2 × 2 × 1 cm) and featureless (Rodriguez et al, 1988; Fleischer et al, 1990), whereas the normal ovaries of a premenopausal woman can range up to 5 × 3 × 2 cm or 10 cm³; the normal postmenopausal woman's ovaries should not measure over 8 cm³ (Cohen, 1989).

Other Pelvic Structures

TVS can depict several other pelvic structures in addition to the uterus and ovaries (Fig. 2-7). These include bowel loops within the pelvis, iliac vessels, and, occasionally, distended fallopian tubes. Even small amounts (1 to 3 mL) of intraperitoneal fluid can be detected in the cul-de-sac or surrounding the uterus.

As mentioned previously, the major pelvic vessels appear as relatively straight tubular structures that course obliquely on either pelvic sidewall. The internal

iliac arteries have a typical width of 5 to 7 mm and tend to pulsate with expansion of both walls, whereas the iliac vein is larger (approximately 1 cm) but does not demonstrate this pulsation. Occasionally, low-level blood echoes will be seen streaming within the vein. The transducer can be manipulated or pivoted to demonstrate these vessels in their long axis. Occasionally a distended distal ureter may have this appearance but not demonstrate pulsations. In most patients, the larger branches of the uterine vessels will be demonstrable by TVS as tubular structures coursing in the paracervical area.

The nondistended fallopian tube is difficult to depict on TVS, probably because of its small intraluminal size and serpiginous course. Occasionally one can identify the origin of the tubes by finding the invagination of endometrium depicting the area of the tubal ostia and following these structures laterally in the axial or coronal plane. The ovarian and infundibulopelvic ligaments usually cannot be depicted.

Sonographic delineation of the tubes is facilitated by intraperitoneal fluid that may be present in the cul-de-sac (Timor-Tritsch and Rottem, 1987). By placing the patient in a reverse-Trendelenburg position, the fluid can be collected around the tube. When surrounded by fluid, the normal tube appears as a 1-cm tubular echogenic structure that usually courses from the lateral aspect of the uterine cornu posterolaterally into the adnexal regions and cul-de-sac. In some patients flaring of the fimbriated end of the tube can be seen, since it approximates its nearby ovary. Transvaginal depiction of the tube is also facilitated when it contains intraluminal fluid.

The transvaginal appearance of the round ligaments is somewhat similar to that arising from a nondistended tube except that their course is straighter and more parallel to the uterine cornu.

Bowel is typically recognized as a fusiform structure frequently containing intraluminal fluid and changes in configuration due to active peristalsis. If there is fluid within the lumen, periotic intraluminal projections resulting from the valvulae conniventes can be seen from small bowel, as can the haustral indentations that are characteristic of large bowel.

Summary

Transvaginal sonography affords detailed depiction of the uterus and ovaries. It requires systematic evaluation of these pelvic structures for their complete delineation in light of the limited field of view of transvaginal transducer probes. An understanding of the anatomic relationship of these structures gained from previous experience with transabdominal sonography, combined

(text continues on page 31)

FIGURE 2-6 Ovaries and Fallopian Tubes

2-6A Left ovary containing a mature follicle. The proximal portion of the left tube is also seen.

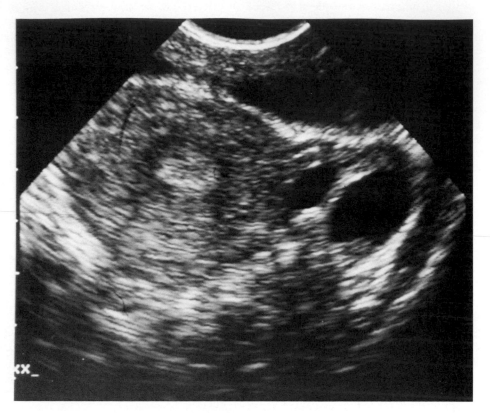

UTERUS   MATURE FOLLICLE

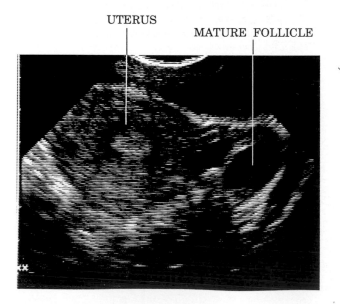

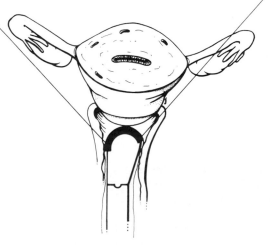

FIGURE 2-6   Ovaries and Fallopian Tubes *(continued)*

2-6B   Right ovary containing an involuted corpus luteum.

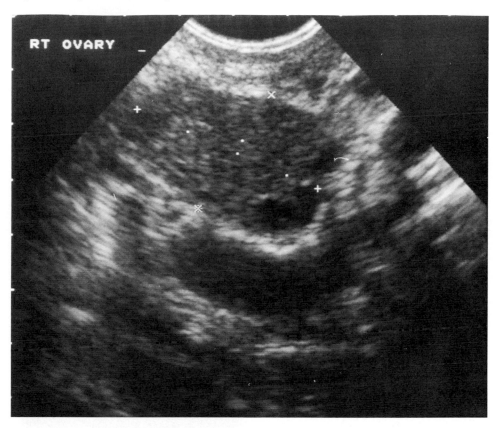

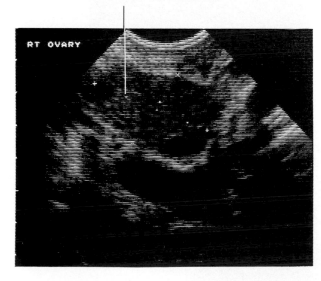

INVOLUTED CORPUS LUTEUM

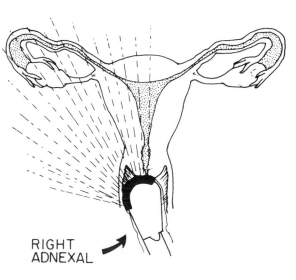

RIGHT
ADNEXAL

(continued)

FIGURE 2-6   **Ovaries and Fallopian Tubes** *(continued)*

2-6C   Normal distal right tube lying in the cul-de-sac. The hysterosalpinogram showed a normally patent tube.

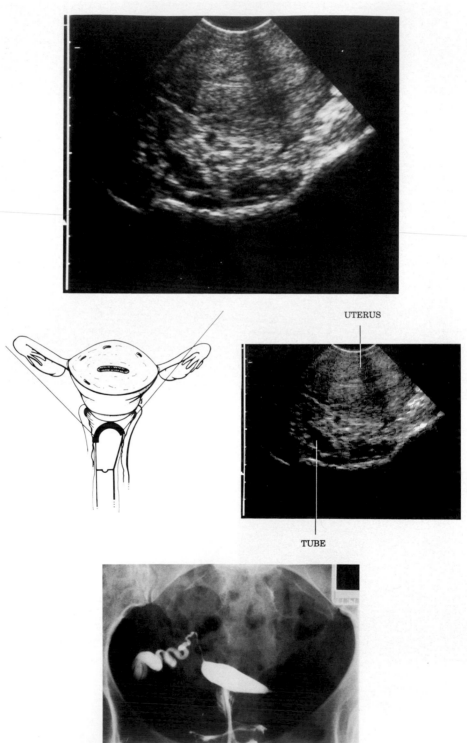

FIGURE 2-7   Bowel

2-7A   Fluid-filled loop of small bowel adjacent to the right overy.

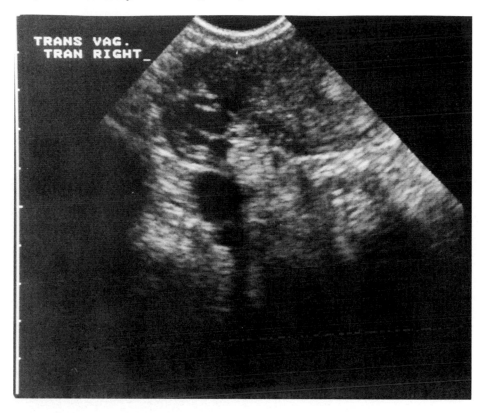

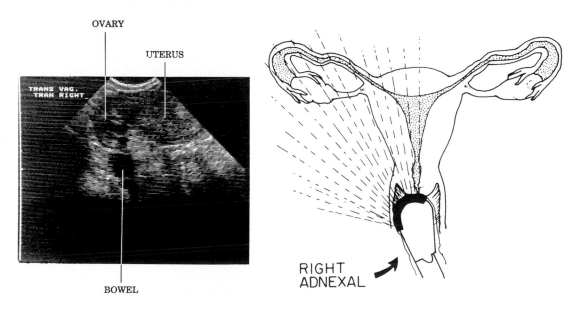

(continued)

FIGURE 2-7   Bowel *(continued)*

2-7B   Large bowel partially filled with feces adjacent to the uterus.

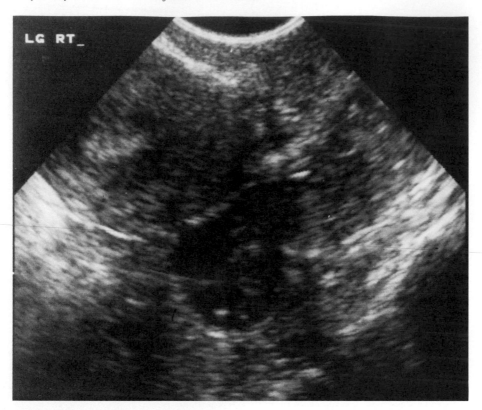

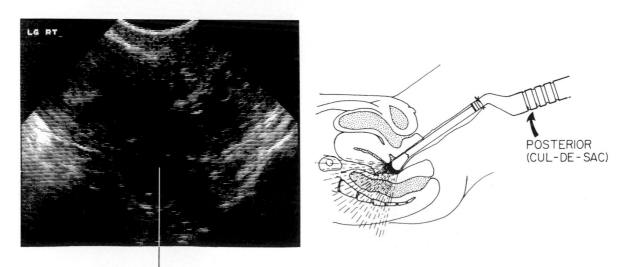

LARGE BOWEL WITH FECES

POSTERIOR
(CUL-DE-SAC)

with the anticipated findings from previous palpation of these structures during a pelvic examination are necessary.

References

Cohen H. The normal size of the ovary: it's bigger than we think. *Radiology* 1989;173(suppl):142.

Fleischer AC, Gordon A, McKee M, et al. Transvaginal sonography of postmenopausal ovaries with pathologic correlation. *J Ultrasound Med* 1990;9:637–640.

Fleischer AC, Mendelson E, Bohm-Velez M. Sonographic depiction of the endometrium with transabdominal and transvaginal scanning. *Semin Ultrasound CT MRI* 1988; 9:81–90.

Granberg S, Wikland M. Comparison between endovaginal and transabdominal transducers for measuring ovarian volume. *J Ultrasound Med* 1987;16:649–654.

Rodriguez M, Platt L, Medearis A, Lacarra M, Lobo R. The use of transvaginal sonography for evaluation of postmenopausal ovarian size and morphology. *Am J Obstet Gynecol* 1988;159:810.

Timor-Tritsch IE, Rottem S. Transvaginal ultrasonographic study of the Fallopian tube. *Obstet Gynecol* 1987;70:424–428.

Chapter *3*

Differential Diagnosis of Pelvic Masses

Arthur C. Fleischer, MD

Introduction

Transvaginal sonography (TVS) is particularly suited for evaluation of patients with pelvic masses of 10 cm or less that lie in the true pelvis. For larger pelvic masses, TVS has only an adjunctive role to transabdominal sonography (TAS). The added definition of the size, location, and internal consistency of pelvic masses afforded by TVS makes it the imaging modality of choice for most pelvic masses (Coleman et al, 1988; Fleischer et al, 1989; Mendleson et al, 1988; Tessler et al, 1989; Andolf and Jorgensen, 1990; Lande et al, 1988; Vilaro, 1987).

The clinically pertinent features of a pelvic mass depicted by TVS include its size and location (ovarian, uterine, or other); its internal consistency (totally cystic, low level echoes, septations, papillary projections, fat, calcifications); and its associated abnormalities (intraperitoneal fluid).

Rather than classifying masses into cystic, complex, and solid categories with conventional TAS, transvaginal sonography affords a more specific differential diagnosis based on more precise delineation, such as the location and internal consistency of the mass. This discussion will reflect a more specific classification afforded by TVS than was possible previously with conventional TAS. Table 3-1 provides a guide for differential diagnosis of pelvic masses using primarily TVS as an adjunct to transabdominal scanning. The following discussion is presented according to these major categories.

Ovarian Masses

Masses that are confined to the ovary typically demonstrate a rim of ovarian tissue surrounding the abnormal lesion. In some cases immature follicles appear as hypoechoic structures within the ovarian parenchyma that help identify the tissue surrounding a mass as ovarian.

The ovary is the site of a variety of pelvic masses, ranging from physiologic cysts to malignant ovarian carcinoma (Figs. 3-1 to 3-5). It is the site of not only primary tumors but also metastatic lesions from gastrointestinal and breast primaries. It can also be the site of tumor sequestration in patients with leukemia.

Physiologic cysts are typically larger than 3 cm and are anechoic, smooth-walled structures. Luteal cysts have a thicker wall than hydropic follicles. Either may contain low-level echoes arising from internal hemorrhage.

Ovarian epithelial tumors tend to demonstrate septae with or without solid areas. Mucinous cystadenomas typically have thin internal septations, whereas serous cystadenomas may be unilocular. Mucinous tumors may contain internal echogenic material arising from the mucin.

Malignant tumors tend to have irregular walls, papillary excrescences, or both. If tumor has spread beyond the capsule, intraperitoneal fluid is usually present as well. Other sonographic features that suggest malignancy include irregularly thick wall or septae and internal solid areas.

Dermoid cysts have a variety of sonographic appearances ranging from anechoic to solid lesions containing echogenic sebum. The anechoic dermoids tend to be encountered in young girls and have a neuroectoderm lining. Dermoids that contain sebum, hair follicles, or both demonstrate echogenic internal material. In some cases the sebum collects anteriorly.

Solid tumors of the ovary may represent primary tumors, metastases, or benign lesions such as fibromas. Hemorrhage may appear as a solid area within an ovary, and these ovaries may torse (see Fig. 3-5). Ovarian torsion should be suspected when an enlarged ovary usually associated with intraperitoneal fluid is seen in a

32

Table 3-1 Differential Diagnoses of Pelvic Masses by TVS

| Location | Consistency | | |
	Cystic	*Complex*	*Solid*
Ovarian	Physiologic cysts Neoplastic cysts	Dermoid cysts Neoplastic cysts Hemorrhagic cysts Tubo-ovarian abscess	Metastases Primary ovarian tumors Fibroma
Adnexal Extraovarian	Paraovarian cysts, hydrosalpinx		Tubal tumor
Uterine			Pedunculated fibroid
Other		Arteriovenous malformation	Bowel tumor, lymphadenopathy

patient with pelvic pain. Color Doppler sonography may be used to definitively confirm the presence of ovarian torsion by the lack of flow to the ovary (Fleischer et al, 1990).

Adnexal Extraovarian Masses

Adnexal extraovarian masses arise from adnexal structures outside the ovary. These include masses such as paraovarian cysts and endometriomas, which can typically be identified as separate from the ovary itself (Fig. 3-6).

Endometriomas have a spectrum of sonographic appearances, ranging from anechoic to echogenic depending on the extent of clot and organization within them. Typically, however, these masses have internal echoes combined with excellent through transmission, indicating that they are predominantly cystic in consistency.

Paraovarian cysts are structures arising from the wolffian duct remnant in the mesovarium. These have similar appearances to peritoneal inclusion cysts, which may arise as a sequela from intraperitoneal surgery. Peritoneal inclusion cysts form from fluid accumulation that is walled off and becomes localized to surrounding serosal structures.

Occasionally tubal masses appear as extraovarian cystic structures. When a tube becomes maximally distended, it is difficult to distinguish it from an ovarian mass. When it is only moderately distended, however, its continuity with the region of the uterine cornu can be established, thus identifying it as a tubal structure.

Solid masses that are extraovarian may on rare occasions represent pedunculated fibroids or tubal carcinoma. In pedunculated fibroids, the sonographer can usually maneuver the probe between the mass and the uterus, showing the pedicle of the pedunculated fibroid. Tubal carcinoma is extremely rare, but it appears as a solid fusiform mass adjacent to the uterus and ovary.

Uterine Masses

The most common uterine mass is the leiomyoma (Fig. 3-7). These masses may simulate the appearance of a pelvic mass if they become subserosal and pedunculated. Usually, however, the intrauterine location of these masses can be established by using the landmarks of the endometrium and applying a small amount of pressure to the uterus to displace the pedicle of a pedunculated fibroid from the uterus proper.

Other Masses

Masses arising from a bowel may on rare occasions appear as pelvic structures (Fig. 3-8). Inflamed terminal ileum and bowel tumors appear as fusiform solid structures usually distinguishable from the uterus and ovary by transvaginal sonography. Diverticulosis appears as a multilayered fusiform structure with punctate hypoechoic areas arising from the diverticula themselves.

Pelvic vessels sometimes may appear as a true mass. Color Doppler sonography can establish the vascular nature of these masses and the presence or absence of arteriovenous fistulae or varices.

Summary

TVS provides important information regarding the size, location, and internal consistency of pelvic masses. Using these parameters and combining the information with clinical data enables TVS to provide a relatively specific diagnosis. More extensive experience and larger studies will assist in evaluating the efficacy of TVS as a means for early detection of ovarian tumors and other pathologic gynecologic disorders.

References

Andolf A, Jorgensen C. A prospective comparison of transabdominal and transvaginal ultrasound with surgical findings in gynecologic disease. *J Ultrasound Med* 1990;9:71–75.

Coleman BG, Arger PH, Grumbach K, et al. Transvaginal and transabdominal sonography: prospective comparison. *Radiology* 1988;168:639–643.

Fleischer A, Gordon A, Entman S. Transabdominal and transvaginal sonography of pelvic masses. *J Ultrasound Med Biol* 1989;15:529–533.

Fleischer A, Rao B, Kepple D. Transvaginal color Doppler sonography: preliminary experience. *Dynamic Cardiovasc Imaging* 1990;3:52–58.

Lande IM, Hill JC, Cosco FE, Kator NN. Adnexal and cul-de-sac abnormalities: transvaginal sonography. *Radiology* 1988;166:325–332.

Mendelson EB, Bohm-Velez M, Joseph N, Neiman HL. Gynecologic imaging: comparison of transabdominal and transvaginal sonography. *Radiology* 1988;66:321–324.

Tessler F, Perrella R, Fleischer A, Grant E. Endovaginal sonography of dilated fallopian tubes. *AJR* 1989;153:523–525.

Vilaro MM, Rifkin MD, Pennell RG, et al. Endovaginal ultrasound: a technique for evaluation of nonfollicular pelvic masses. *J Ultrasound Med* 1987;6:697–701.

FIGURE 3-1   Cystic Ovarian Masses

3-1A   TAS showing an anechoic right adnexal mass (between cursors).

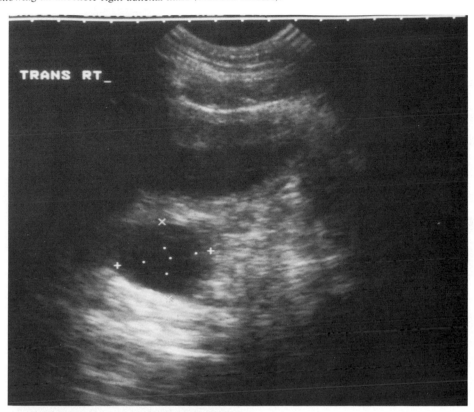

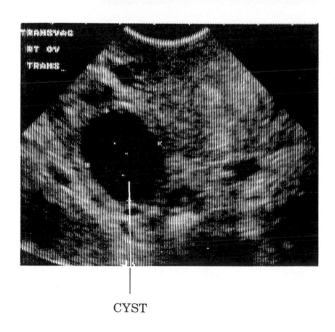

CYST

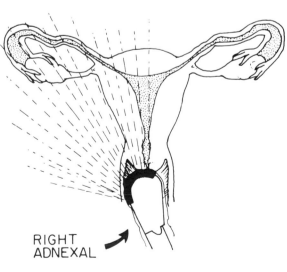

RIGHT
ADNEXAL

(continued)

FIGURE 3-1   Cystic Ovarian Masses *(continued)*

3-1B   TVS of same patient in 3-1*A* demonstrating the cyst (between cursors) within the compressed residual ovarian tissue (arrow).

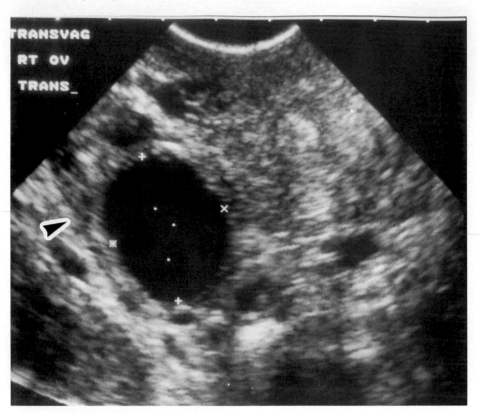

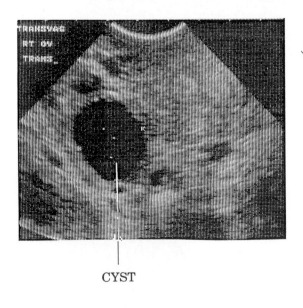

CYST

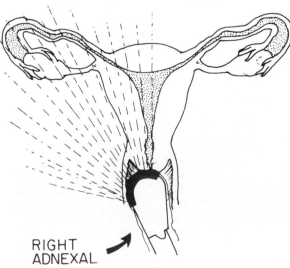

RIGHT
ADNEXAL

FIGURE 3-1   Cystic Ovarian Masses *(continued)*

3-1C   TVS of a hemorrhagic corpus luteum containing multiple thin synchae.

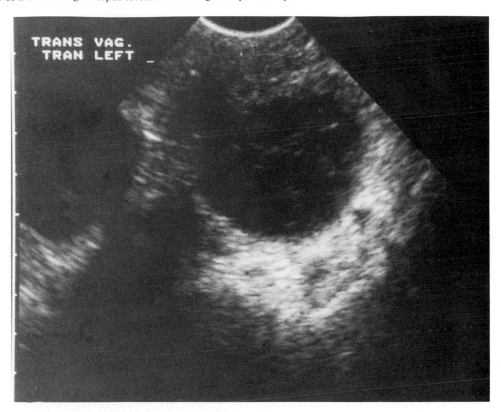

HEMORRHAGIC CORPUS LUTEUM

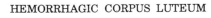

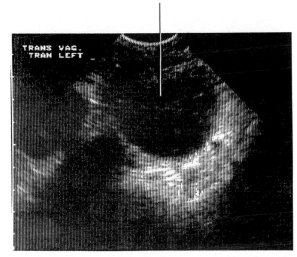

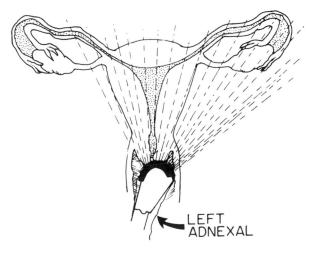

LEFT ADNEXAL

FIGURE 3-2   Septated Ovarian Masses

3-2A   TVS of mucinous cystadenoma (between cursors) with multiple septae.

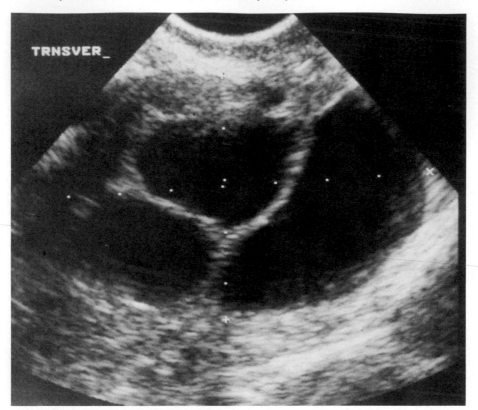

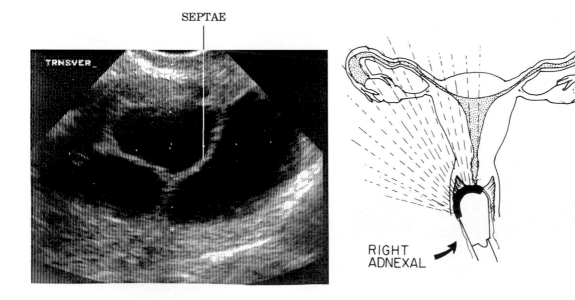

FIGURE 3-2   Septated Ovarian Masses *(continued)*

3-2B   TVS of bilateral cystadenomas (between cursors) with numerous septae.

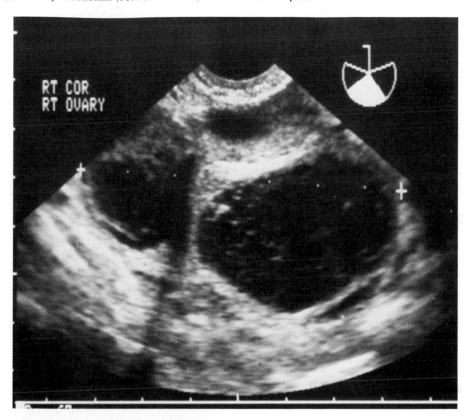

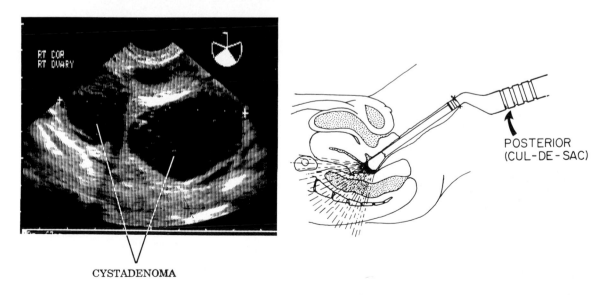

CYSTADENOMA

POSTERIOR
(CUL-DE-SAC)

(continued)

FIGURE 3-2 **Septated Ovarian Masses** *(continued)*

3-2C TVS of an 8 × 12 cm complex mass containing septae and solid material. This was a hemorrhagic ovarian cyst.

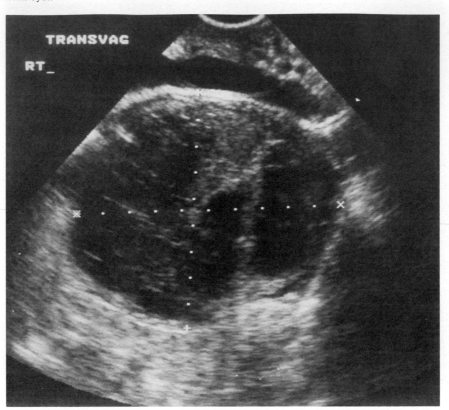

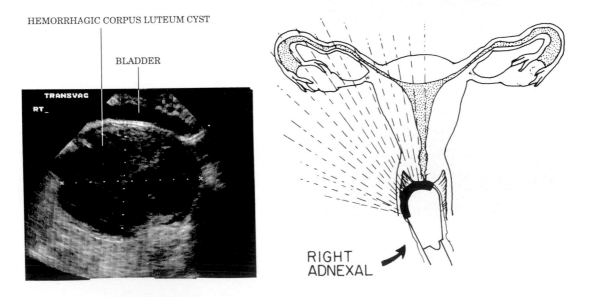

FIGURE 3-3   Cystic Ovarian Mass Containing Solid Elements

3-3A   TVS of metastases from gastrointestinal primary containing papillary excrescences.

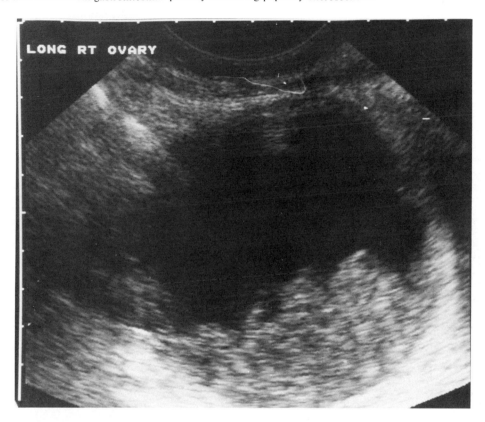

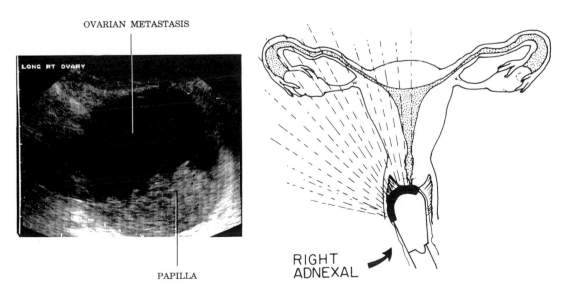

OVARIAN METASTASIS

PAPILLA

RIGHT
ADNEXAL

(continued)

FIGURE 3-3   Cystic Ovarian Mass Containing Solid Elements *(continued)*

3-3B   TVS of an endometrioid carcinoma containing an irregular solid area.

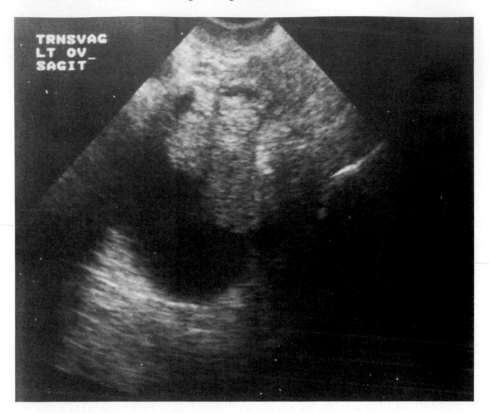

SOLID AREA

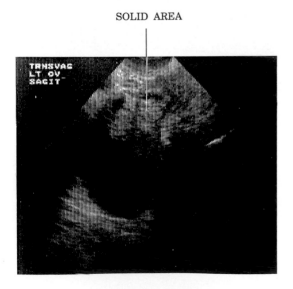

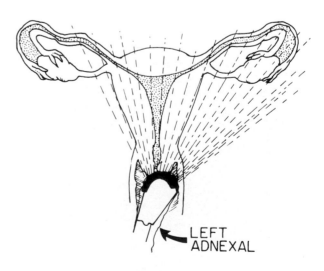

LEFT ADNEXAL

FIGURE 3-4   **Complex Adnexal Masses**

3-4A   TVS of a dermoid cyst containing a layer of sebum.

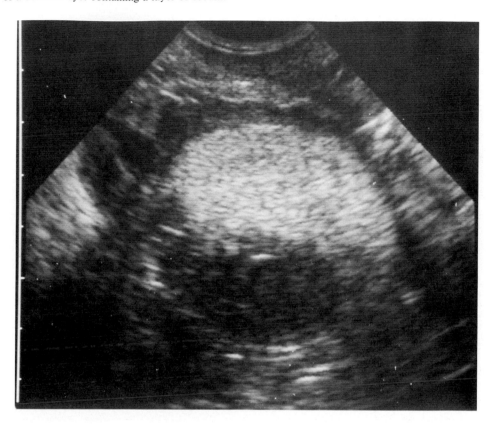

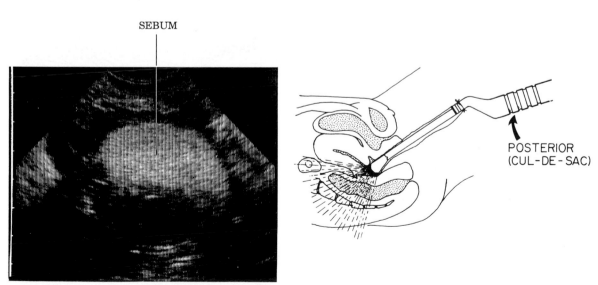

SEBUM

POSTERIOR
(CUL-DE-SAC)

(continued)

FIGURE 3-4   Complex Adnexal Masses *(continued)*

3-4B   Dermoid cyst that is difficult to delineate due to echogenic interfaces created by hair and fat.

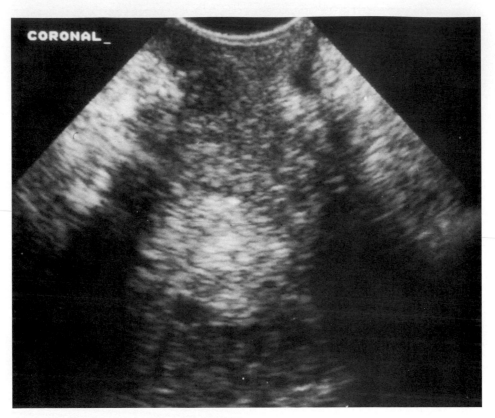

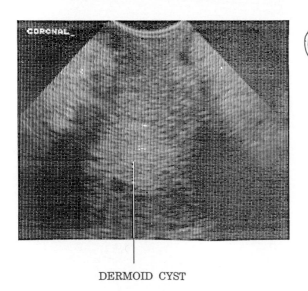

DERMOID CYST

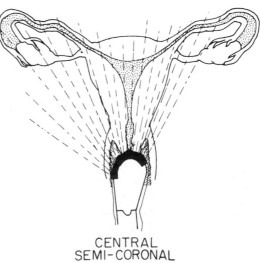

CENTRAL
SEMI-CORONAL

FIGURE 3-4   Complex Adnexal Masses *(continued)*

3-4C   Sectioned dermoid cyst that appeared on TVS as in *B*.

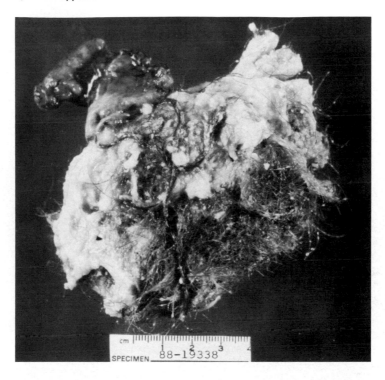

FIGURE 3-5   Solid Ovarian Masses

3-5A   TVS of an endometrioma adjacent to a follicle-containing right ovary. The endometrioma appears solid due to the original clot it contains.

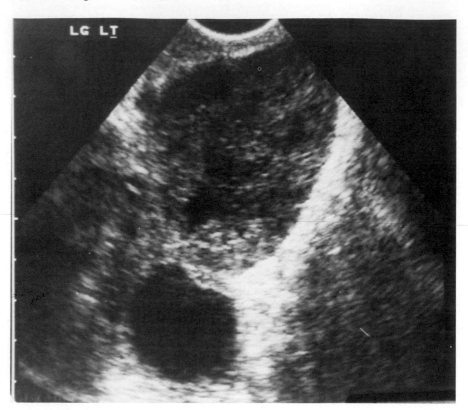

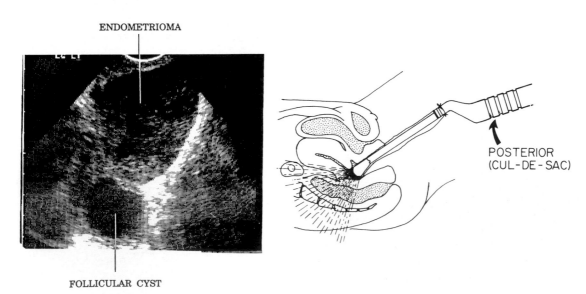

FIGURE 3-5   **Solid Ovarian Masses** *(continued)*

3-5B   TVS of a solid ovarian mass containing fibrous strands resulting from extensive
hemorrhage within the left ovary.

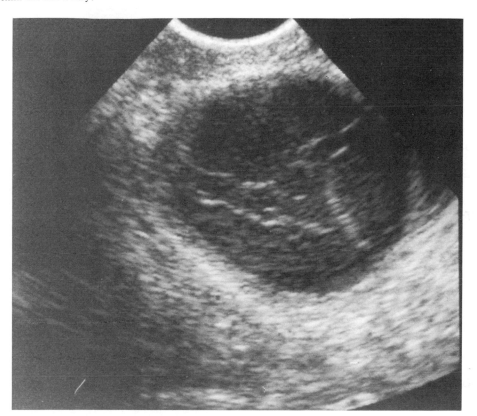

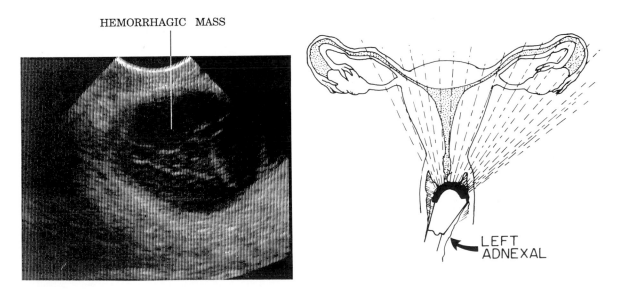

HEMORRHAGIC   MASS

LEFT
ADNEXAL

FIGURE 3-6   Adnexal Extraovarian Masses

3-6A   TVS of a paraovarian cyst separate from the ovary.

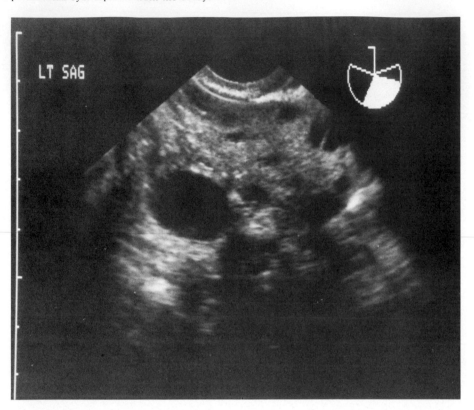

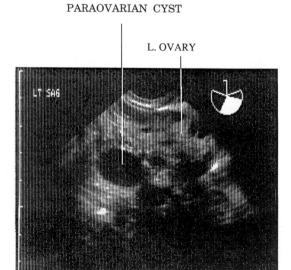

PARAOVARIAN CYST

L. OVARY

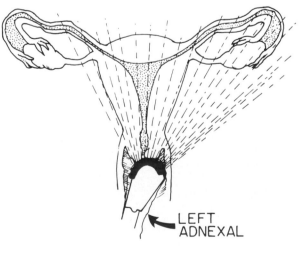

FIGURE 3-6   Adnexal Extraovarian Masses *(continued)*

3-6B   TVS of an endometrioma containing echogenic material that layered posteriorly, representing clotted blood.

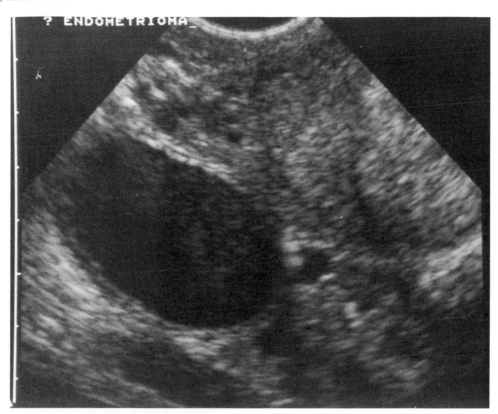

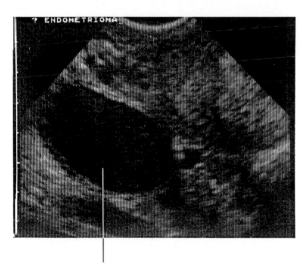

BLOOD WITHIN ENDOMETRIOMA

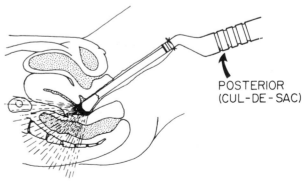

POSTERIOR
(CUL-DE-SAC)

(continued)

FIGURE 3-6   **Adnexal Extraovarian Masses** *(continued)*

3-6C   TVS of a large hydrosalpinx (between cursors) appearing as a fusiform cystic
structure posterior to the uterus.

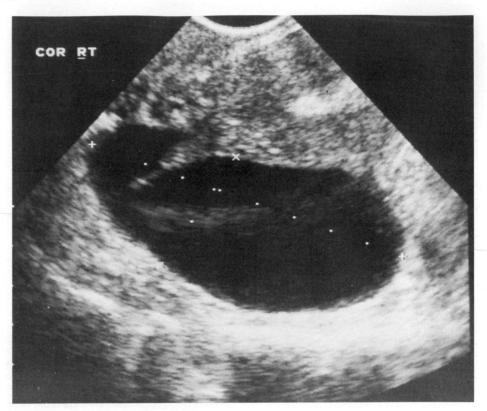

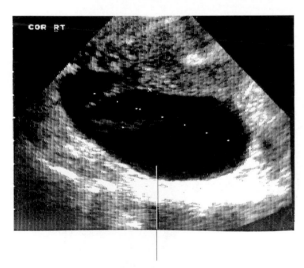

HYDROSALPINX

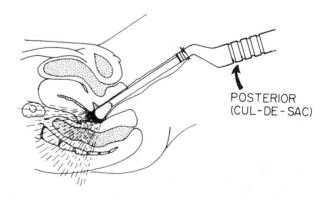

POSTERIOR
(CUL-DE-SAC)

FIGURE 3-6 Adnexal Extraovarian Masses *(continued)*

3-6D Endometrioma containing clotted blood and formed clot.

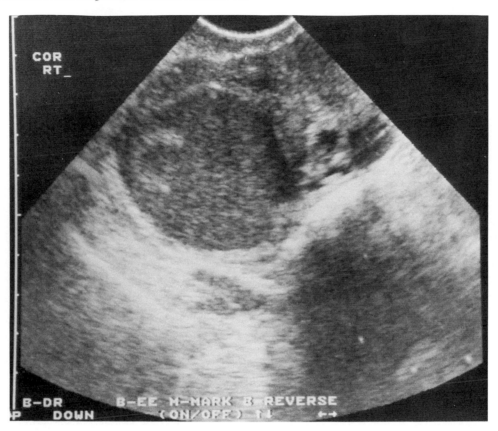

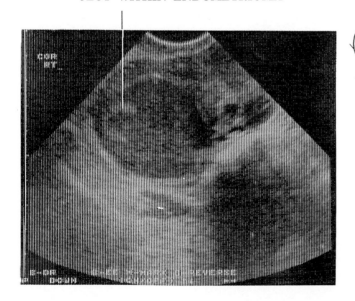

CLOT WITHIN ENDOMETRIOMA

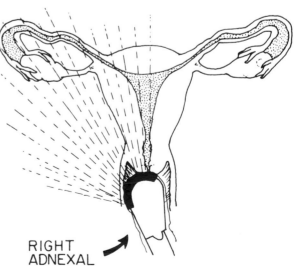

RIGHT
ADNEXAL

(continued)

FIGURE 3-6   Adnexal Extraovarian Masses *(continued)*

3-6E   Large endometrioma containing clotted blood. Note excellent through transmission, indicating fluid contents of mass.

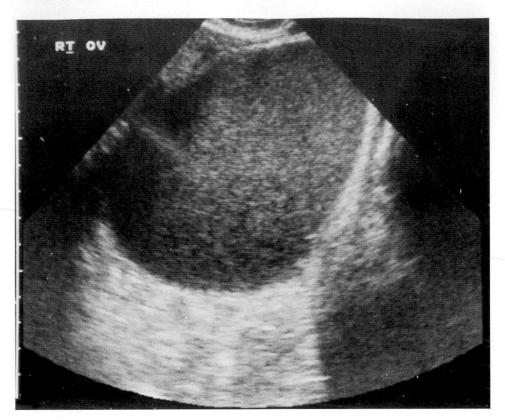

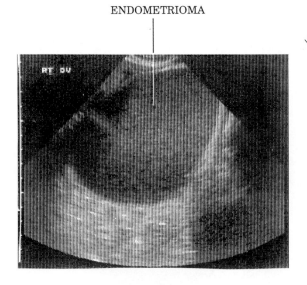

ENDOMETRIOMA

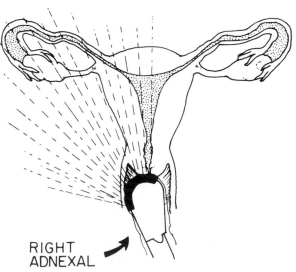

RIGHT ADNEXAL

FIGURE 3-7 Uterine Masses

3-7A TVS of large solid pelvic mass (between cursors). It was difficult to determine the origin of the mass in TVS.

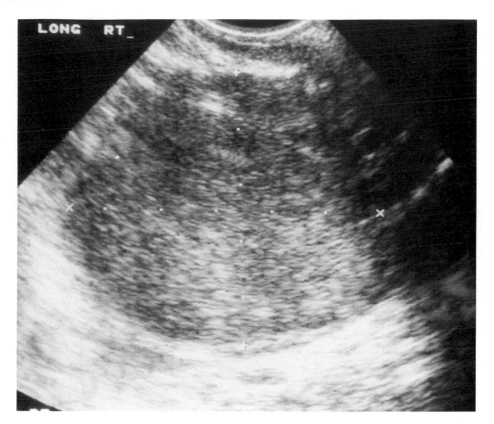

SOLID MASS

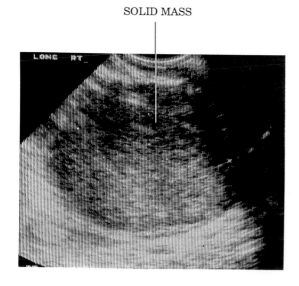

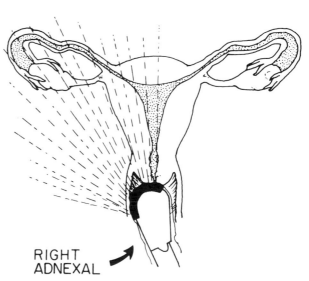

RIGHT
ADNEXAL

(continued)

FIGURE 3-7   Uterine Masses *(continued)*

3-7B   TAS of the same patient as in *A* showing that the fibroid (between cursors) arises from the posterior corpus of the uterus.

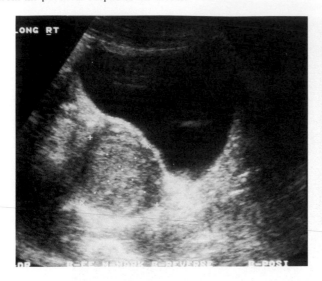 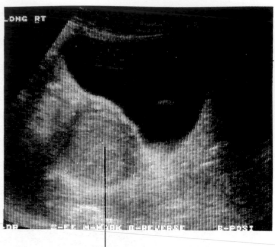

FIBROID

FIGURE 3-7 Uterine Masses *(continued)*

3-7C TVS of intramural fibroid (between cursors). The position of the fibroid relative to the endometrium is shown.

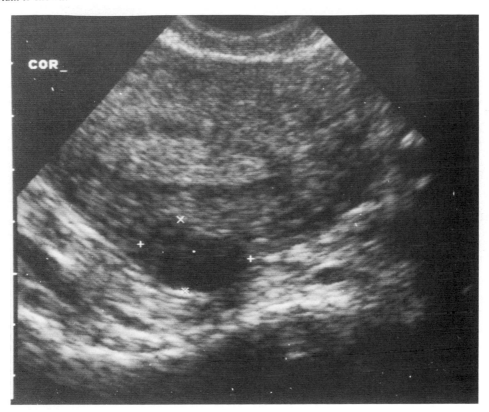

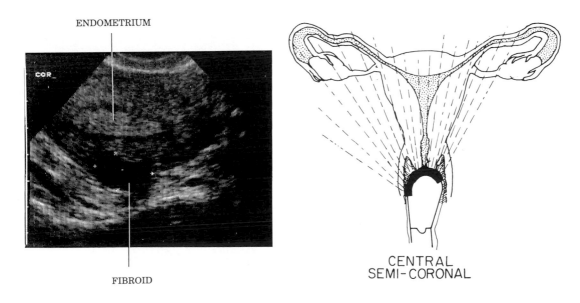

FIGURE 3-8   Other Pelvic Masses

3-8A   TVS of a thickened loop of small bowel in a patient with Crohn's disease.

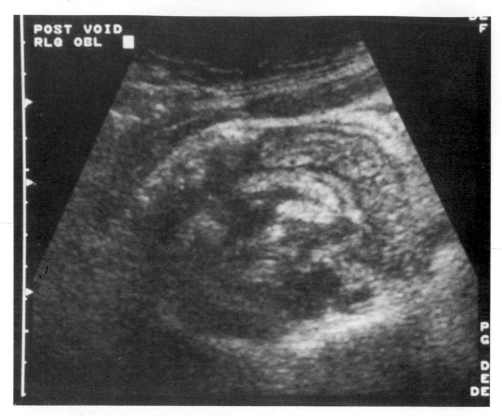

ABNORMAL TERMINAL ILEUM

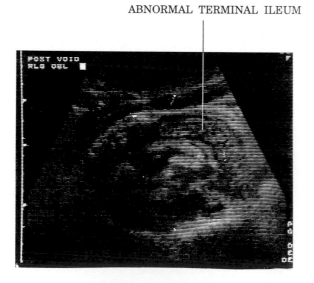

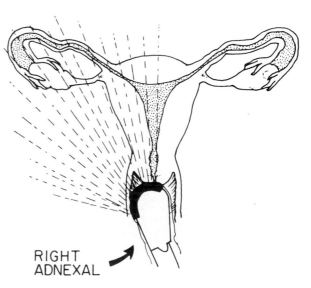

RIGHT ADNEXAL

FIGURE 3-8   Other Pelvic Masses *(continued)*

3-8B   TVS of a markedly thickened bowel loop in a patient with advanced Crohn's disease.

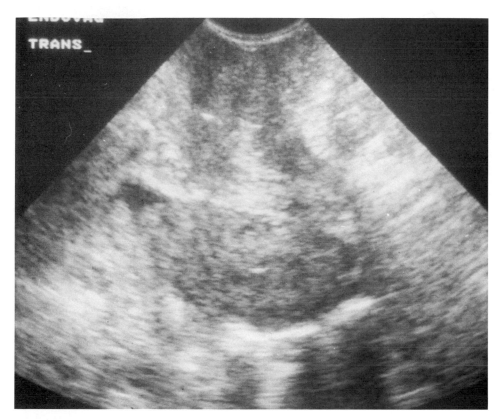

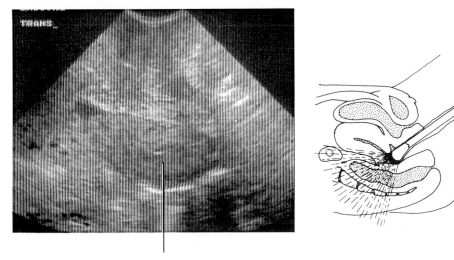

BOWEL MASS

POSTERIOR
(CUL-DE-SAC)

(continued)

FIGURE 3-8 Other Pelvic Masses *(continued)*

3-8C Diverticulosis of sigmoid colon appearing as multilayered fusiform structure.

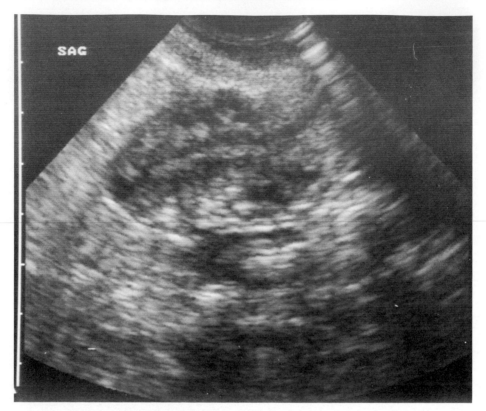

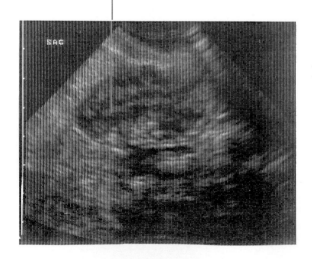

SIGMOID DIVERTICULOSIS

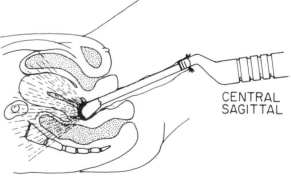

CENTRAL SAGITTAL

FIGURE 3-8   Other Pelvic Masses *(continued)*

3-8D   Radiograph taken from barium enema of patient in *C* showing diverticulosis of sigmoid colon.

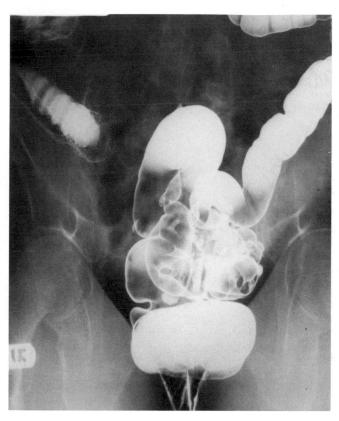

Chapter 4

Uterine Disorders

Arthur C. Fleischer, MD
Donna M. Kepple, RDMS

Introduction

Transvaginal sonography (TVS) affords detailed delineation of the uterus and its myometrium, endometrium, and vessels (Mendelson et al, 1988). Because of this, several uterine disorders may be evaluated by TVS. After discussion of normal anatomy and scanning technique, this chapter will discuss the use of TVS in the evaluation of a variety of both benign and malignant uterine disorders. The potential applications of transvaginal color Doppler sonography will also be presented.

Normal Anatomy and Scanning Technique

The uterus can be imaged in three major scanning planes with TVS. These include views in its long axis, an oblique semicoronal or semiaxial plane, and a short-axis view (Fig. 4-1A to C). The long-axis image is obtained when the transducer-probe is introduced into the vagina and the uterus is imaged in the greatest long axis. The semicoronal depiction of the uterus is obtained when the transducer is turned 90 degrees to the long axis and imaged in its greatest longitudinal plane. For anteflexed uteri, the probe handle is held posteriorly with the beam directed anteriorly; the opposite maneuver is used for retroflexed uteri. In the semicoronal scanning plane, the uterus is imaged in its width. The short-axis view is obtained by retracting the transducer-probe into the mid-vagina and directing it anteriorly through the fornix.

The uterus varies in its size and shape depending on the patient's parity and whether or not the patient is premenopausal or postmenopausal (Table 4-1). TVS should not be attempted until the patient is in her late teens; therefore, the discussion of uterine anatomy will begin in patients that are nulliparous and postpubertal.

The size of the uterus in these patients is approximately 6 cm in length and 3 to 4 cm in the anteroposterior (AP) and transverse dimensions. In the parous patient, the uterine long axis can be up to 8 cm in length, whereas in the postmenopausal woman, the uterus decreases in size to approximately 4 to 6 cm in long axis.

Variations in the normal anatomy of the central endometrial interfaces can be detected in patients who have fusion abnormalities of the uterus (Fig. 4-2A,B). Specifically, the bicornuate uterus can be readily identified by the two echogenic endometrial lumina. Other anatomic variations include prominence of myometrial arcuate vessels and calcification of these vessels in the elderly patient. Small (less than 1 cm) cervical inclusion cysts (nabothian) may be present within the cervix.

The myometrial fibers are arranged in a specific pattern. They provide effective contraction of the uterus in the normal cycle (Lyons et al, 1989). Occasionally a sustained contraction can appear as a hypoechoic rounded area. These contractions can be detected on TVS if the study is recorded and played at fast-forward on a videocassette recorder, and their direction and intensity can be seen. During menses, these contractions begin at the fundus and extend to the cervix. In midcycle, they are propagated in the opposite direction. Perhaps these contractions affect the efficiency of sperm transport, thereby optimizing the chances of implantation.

Blood is supplied to the uterus by the uterine artery, a branch of the hypogastric artery. Arcuate vessels are present in the outer third of the myometrium. The venous structures are more prominent than the arterial ones (see Fig. 4-2B). Triplex color Doppler of these vessels can be obtained to assess the relative uterine perfusion (see Fig. 12-1).

TVS clearly depicts changes in the endometrial texture and thickness during the menstrual cycle (Fig. 4-3). In the menstrual phase, the endometrium appears as an interrupted interface that is thin and has some

Table 4-1 Uterine Size (cm)

	Length	Width	AP	Volume (mL)	Cx: Corpus/ Fundus
Adult (nulliparous)	6–8	3–5	3–5	30–40	1:2
Adult (parous)	8–10	5–6	5–6	60–80	1:2
Postmenopausal	3–5	2–3	2–3	14–17	1:1

From Warwick W, ed. *Gray's Anatomy*, 35th ed. Philadelphia: WB Saunders, 1973:1356.

hypoechoic areas related to extravasated blood and sloughing tissue (see Fig. 4-3A). In the proliferative phase, the endometrium appears as isoechoic to the myometrium (Fig. 4-3B). During the preovulatory phase, the endometrium may have a multilayered appearance with an inner hypoechoic layer and an echogenic outer layer (see Fig. 4-3C). The inner hypoechoic layer probably represents the inner myometrium, which is relatively edematous. In the secretory phase, the thickness measures between 8 and 14 mm, and the endometrium is echogenic (see Fig. 4-3D). This is probably related to mucous and glycogen stored in the endometrial glands and the echogenic interfaces provided by the tortuous glands. Table 4-2 includes the relative thicknesses of the endometrium throughout the cycle. The thickness of the endometrium is given as an endometrial "width" that includes both layers measured in the greatest AP dimension.

Leiomyoma

Leiomyomas are common tumors consisting of smooth muscle and connective tissue arising from the soft tissue and smooth muscle covering the intramyometrial arcuate vessels. They can remain intramural. If they extend into the uterine lumen or submucosa, or extend outward, they become pedunculated and subserosal. Leiomyomas have a variety of sonographic textures, ranging from hypoechoic to echogenic with a calcified

Table 4-2 Endometrial Thickness

	Range (mm)
Proliferative phase	4–8
Secretory phase	7–14
Postmenopausal (no HRT)	4–8
Postmenopausal (HRT)	6–10

HRT, hormone replacement therapy.

border (Fig. 4-4A to C). This is to be expected since these tumors have a varying amount of smooth muscle and connective tissue.

TVS can be used to monitor the size of leiomyomas. Color Doppler sonography may help identify those leiomyomas that are vascular and may be responsive to GnRH analog (Lupron) treatment (Friedman et al, 1987). TVS is particularly helpful in identifying intraligamentous fibroids and the pedicle of pedunculated subserosal fibroids thereby differentiating these from intramural fibroids (see Fig. 4-4C).

Endometrial Hyperplasia

Bleeding in the postmenopausal woman is a fairly common phenomenon, but could be an indicator of endometrial carcinoma. The differential diagnosis includes atrophic endometrium, which is prone to hemorrhagic ulceration or estrogen-induced hyperplasia of the endometrium.

Although there are no large studies at this time that set the upper limits of the thickness of the endometrium in healthy postmenopausal women, it should be thin and atrophic and less than approximately 10 mm in the AP dimension (Fig. 4-5) (Goldstein et al, 1990). It may be slightly thicker than this in patients on hormone replacement therapy.

TVS is used in the evaluation of postmenopausal women who have vaginal bleeding. Endometrial thickening greater than 10 mm in the AP dimension in patients who are postmenopausal usually indicates either hyperplasia or carcinoma (Goldstein et al, 1990). TVS can assess the amount of tissue within the endometrium and is predictive in cases where there is scant (less than 6 mm width) endometrium, but these samples might have insufficient tissue for diagnosis or scant cellular material. The relative amount of tissue that will be retrieved by dilation and curettage can be predicted by the appearance of the endometrium on TVS. Measuring the endometrium in length, AP dimension, and width enables estimation of endometrial volume (Fleischer, 1990).

TVS is not a screening procedure in patients with endometrial hyperplasia, since the evaluation of these patients needs to be based on a histopathologic diagnosis. TVS can supply information concerning the relative amount of endometrial hyperplasia, however. Sonographic images of endometrial thickening may result from hyperplasia but actually represent polyps over 5 to 10 mm. Since these are usually compressed, however, individual polyps may not be discernible with TVS.

TVS may detect thickened endometria in patients being evaluated for an adnexal mass. If the endometrium is over 10 mm in the AP dimension or over 5 to 10 cm^3 in volume, an endometrial biopsy may be indicated, especially if there is a history of bleeding, since hyperplasia is a known precursor to carcinoma (Ferenczy, 1988).

Endometrial Neoplasms

TVS aids in assessment of the depth of invasion in patients with histologically proven endometrial carcinoma (Gordon et al, 1990). The extent of invasion can be detected in most cases and classified as superficial, intermediate, or deep, depending on the extent of the tumor invasion relative to the myometrial thickness ($>50\%$ = deep) (Fig. 4-6A to D) and extension into the cervix (Fig. 4-7).

Most endometrial tumors are echogenic, although less well-differentiated tumors may be hypoechoic (see Fig. 4-6B,C) (Gordon et al, 1990). Difficulties arise in tumors that are exophytic or those that stretch the myometrium but do not invade it. Microscopic invasion is also not detectable, and preexisting conditions such as leiomyoma and adenomyoma may make it difficult to precisely delineate the extent of myometrial invasion.

Other Conditions

TVS can also evaluate patients with suspected adenomyosis. In adenomyosis the sonographic findings range from normal sonographic appearances to echogenic myometrium caused by multiple adenomyomas. Endometritis may also demonstrate an echogenic pattern and thickening of the endometrium.

One should also realize that retained secretions, either mucous or serous, can simulate endometrial pathology.

Summary

TVS is the diagnostic modality of choice for evaluating most uterine disorders. It is particularly useful in identifying the exact location and size of leiomyomas and other uterine tumors.

References

Ferenczy A. Endometrial hyperplasia and neoplasia: a two disease concept. In: Berkowitz RL, Cohen CJ, Kase NG, eds. *Obstetric Ultrasonography/Gynecologic Oncology.* New York: Churchill Livingstone, 1988:197–213.
Fleischer A, Gordon A, Entman S, Kepple D. Transvaginal sonography of the endometrium: current and potential clinical applications. *CRC Crit Rev Diagn Imaging* 1990; 30:85–110.
Friedman AJ, Barbieri RL, Benacerraf BR, Schiff I. Treatment of leiomyomata with intranasal or subcutaneous leuprolide, a gonadotropin-releasing hormone agonist. *Fertil Steril* 1987;48:560–564.
Goldstein SR, Nachtigall M, Snyder JR, Nachtigall L. Endometrial assessment by vaginal ultrasonography before endometrial sampling in patients with postmenopausal bleeding. *Am J Obstet Gynecol* 1990;163:119–123.
Gordon AN, Fleischer AC, Reed GW. Depth of myometrial invasion in endometrial cancer: preoperative assessment by transvaginal ultrasonography. *Gynecol Oncol.* In press.
Warwick W, ed. *Gray's Anatomy,* 35th ed. Philadelphia: WB Saunders, 1973:1356.
Lyons EA, Gallard G, Zheng X-H, Levi CS, Lindsay DJ. Contractions of the inner myometrium in fertility (abstract). *Radiology* 1989;173:114. Abstract.
Mendelson EB, Bohm-Velez M, Joseph N, Neiman HL. Endometrial abnormalities: evaluation with transvaginal sonography. *AJR* 1988;150:139–142.

FIGURE 4-1   Normal Uterus

4-1A   In long axis.

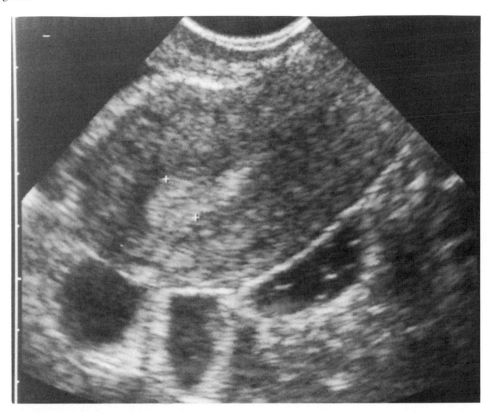

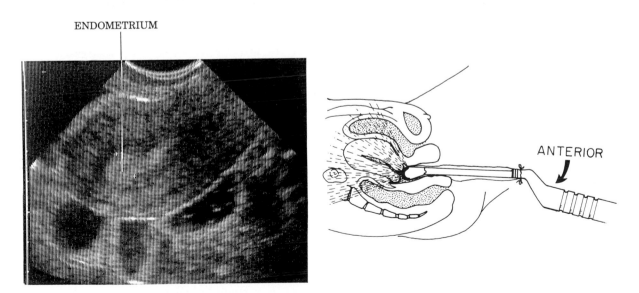

ENDOMETRIUM

ANTERIOR

(continued)

FIGURE 4-1   Normal Uterus *(continued)*

4-1B   In semicoronal plane. Note invagination of endometrium into tubal ostia within uterine cornua.

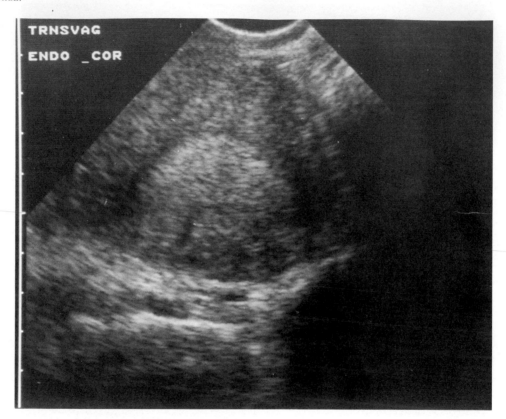

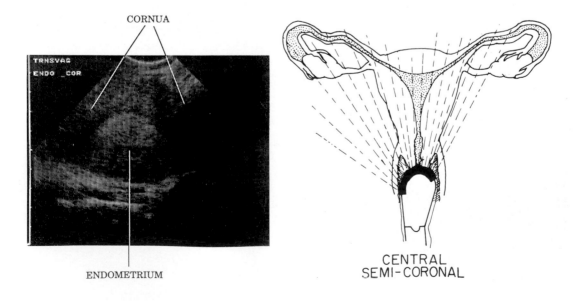

FIGURE 4-1   Normal Uterus *(continued)*

4-1C In short axis showing secretory phase endometrium. Note where endometrium invaginates into area of tubal ostia.

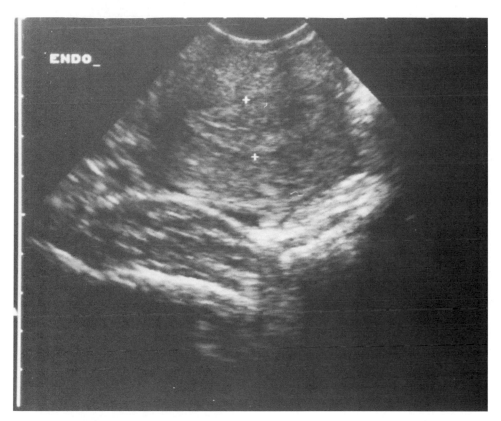

SECRETORY ENDOMETRIUM

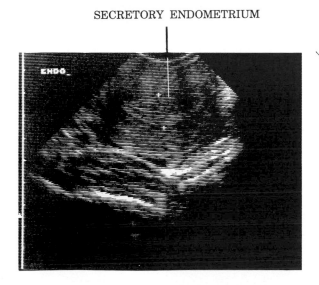
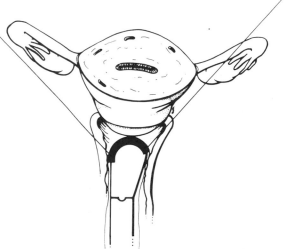

(continued)

FIGURE 4-1   Normal Uterus *(continued)*

4-1D   Retroflexed uterus in long axis.

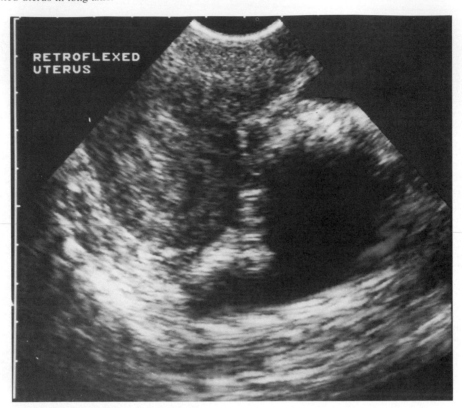

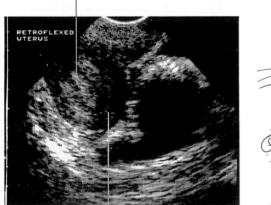

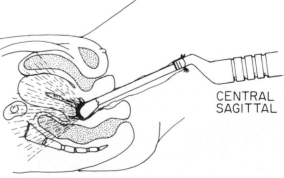

FIGURE 4-1   **Normal Uterus** *(continued)*

4-1E   Normal atrophic endometrium in postmenopausal women.

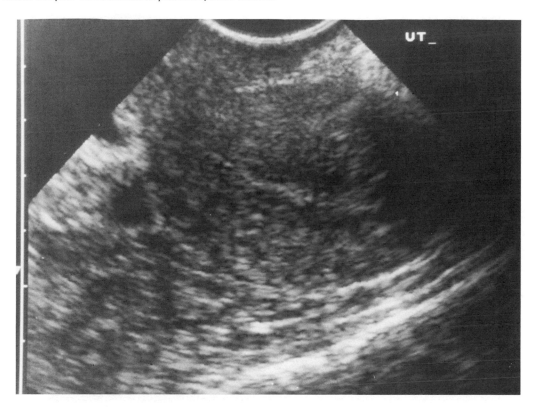

ATROPHIC ENDOMETRIUM

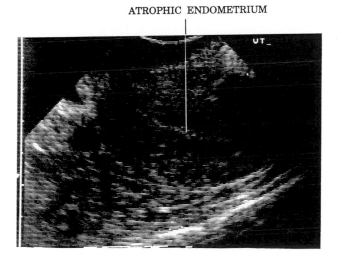

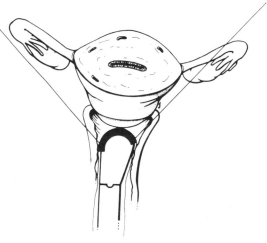

FIGURE 4-2   **Normal Variants**

4-2A   Bicornuate uterus demonstrating two endometria. R, right horn; L, left horn.

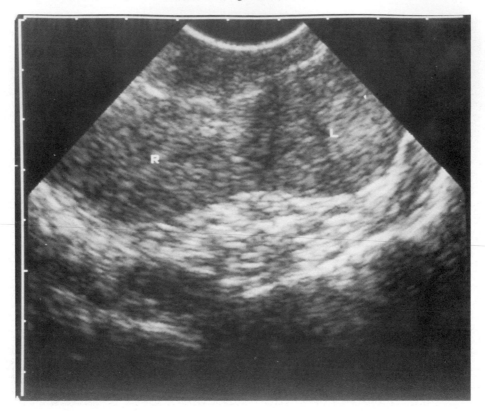

BICORNUATE UTERUS

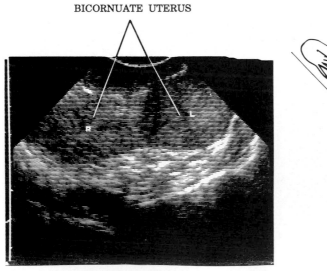

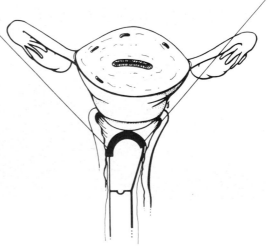

FIGURE 4-2   Normal Variants *(continued)*

4-2B   Same as *A*, in a semicoronal plane showing both endometria.

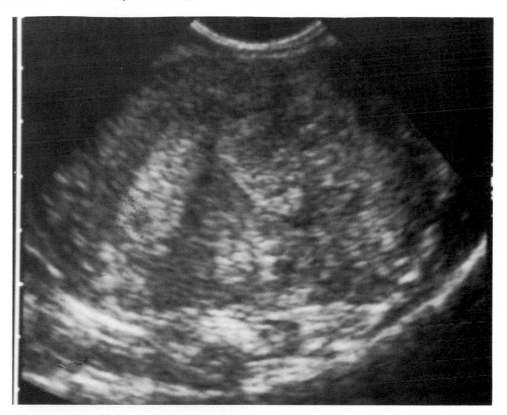

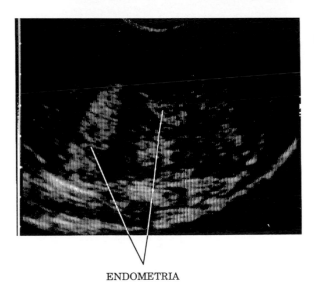

ENDOMETRIA

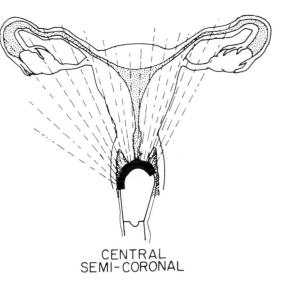

CENTRAL
SEMI-CORONAL

(continued)

FIGURE 4-2 Normal Variants *(continued)*

4-2C Calcifications with arcuate artery in an elderly woman.

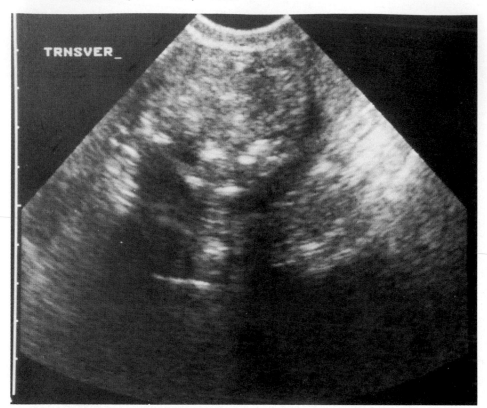

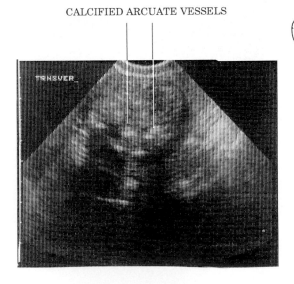

CALCIFIED ARCUATE VESSELS

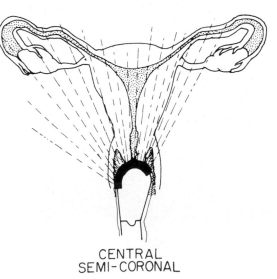

CENTRAL
SEMI-CORONAL

FIGURE 4-3 Endometrial Changes During a Spontaneous Cycle

4-3A Menstrual phase—sloughing of the endometrium and a myometrial contraction. A physiologic amount of cul-de-sac fluid is also present.

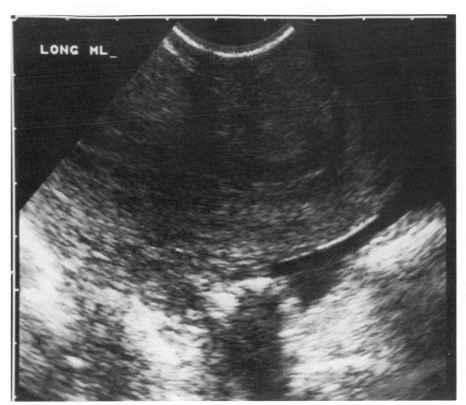

ENDOMETRIUM

CONTRACTION

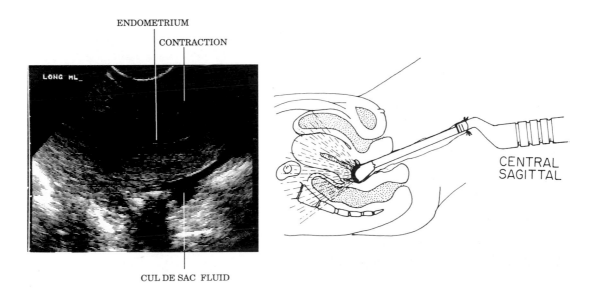

CENTRAL SAGITTAL

CUL DE SAC FLUID

(continued)

FIGURE 4-3   Endometrial Changes During a Spontaneous Cycle *(continued)*

4-3B   Proliferative phase—isoechoic to myometrium.

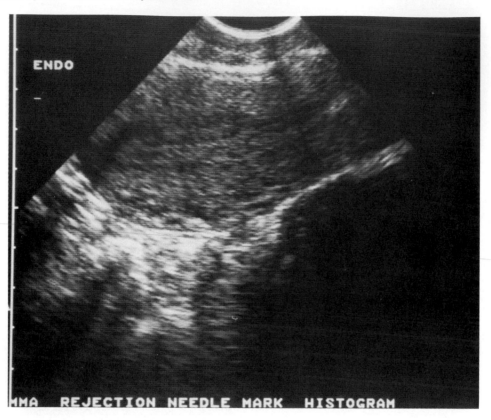

ENDOMETRIUM

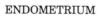

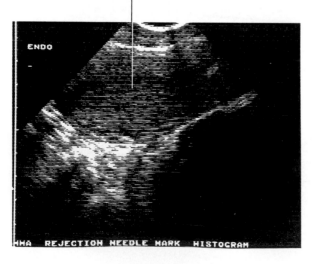

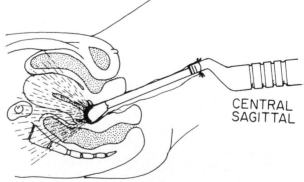

FIGURE 4-3   **Endometrial Changes During a Spontaneous Cycle** *(continued)*

4-3C   Periovulatory period—multiple layers due to edema of the compactum layer.

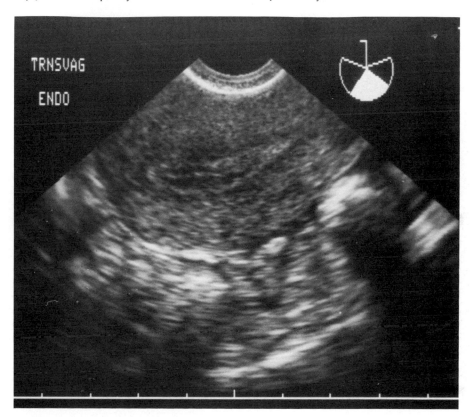

MULTILAYERED ENDOMETRIUM

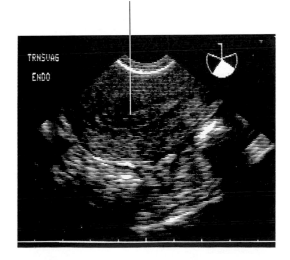

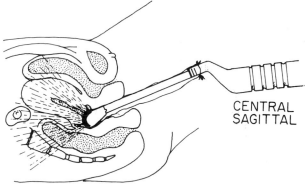

CENTRAL
SAGITTAL

(continued)

FIGURE 4-3   **Endometrial Changes During a Spontaneous Cycle** *(continued)*

4-3D   Secretory phase—echogenic and thick due to mucus and glycogen stored within glands (between cursors).

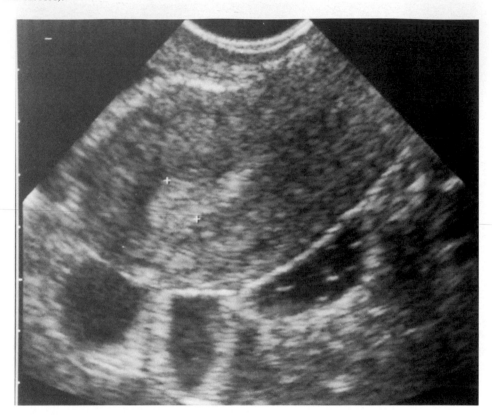

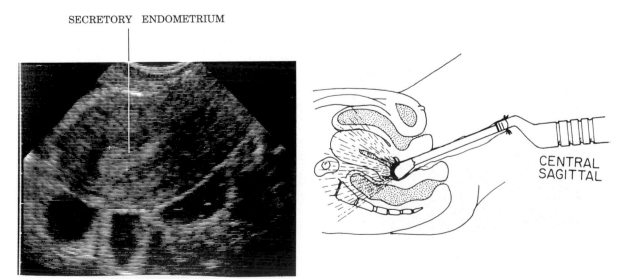

SECRETORY ENDOMETRIUM

CENTRAL SAGITTAL

FIGURE 4-4   Leiomyoma

4-4A   Small hypoechoic intramural fibroid.

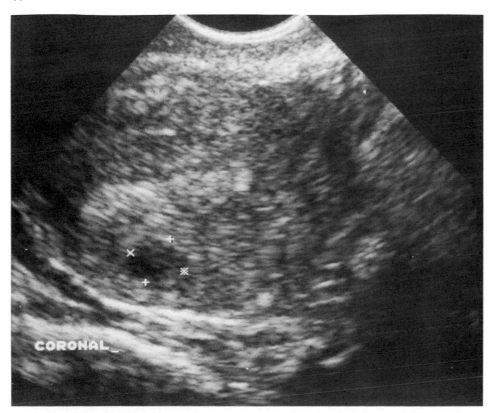

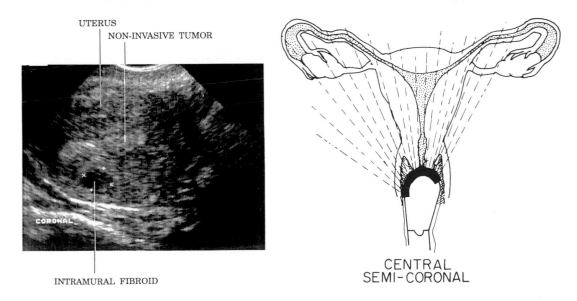

UTERUS

NON-INVASIVE TUMOR

INTRAMURAL FIBROID

CENTRAL
SEMI-CORONAL

(continued)

FIGURE 4-4   Leiomyoma *(continued)*

4-4B   Intramural fibroid separate from the endometrium.

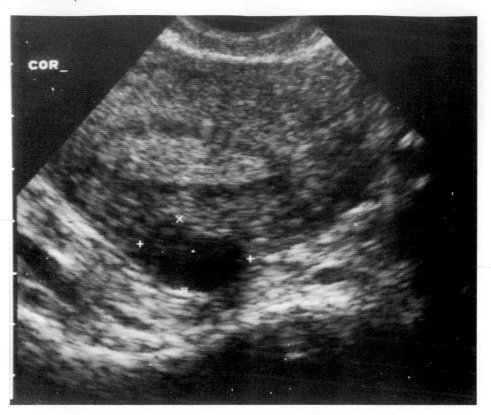

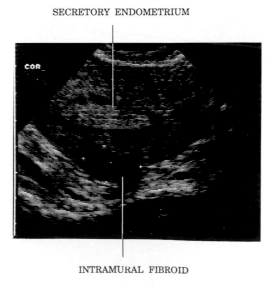

SECRETORY ENDOMETRIUM

INTRAMURAL FIBROID

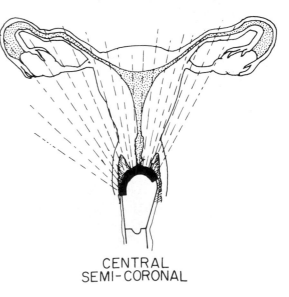

CENTRAL
SEMI-CORONAL

FIGURE 4-4   Leiomyoma *(continued)*

4-4C   Cervical fibroid. TVS (left); sectioned specimen (right).

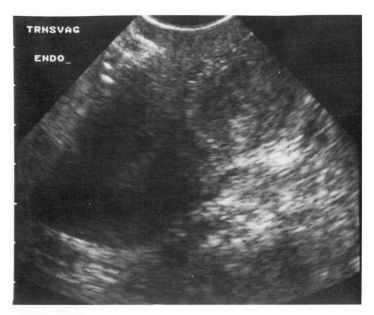

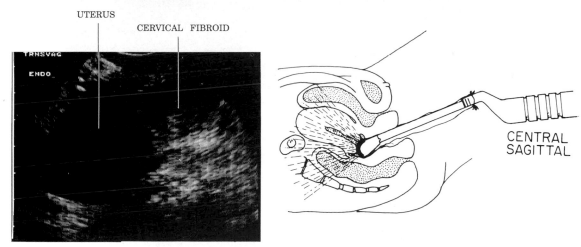

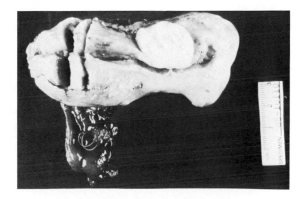

(continued)

FIGURE 4-4   Leiomyoma *(continued)*

4-4D   Submucous fibroid.

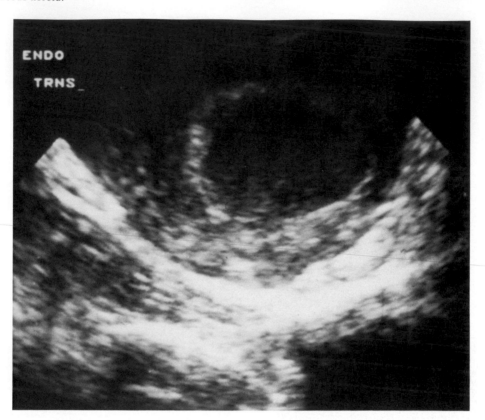

SUBMUCOUSAL FIBROID

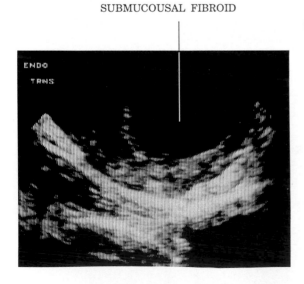

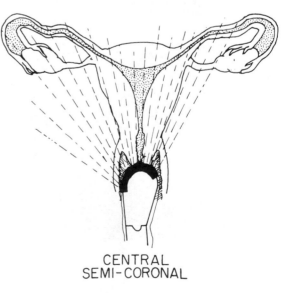

CENTRAL
SEMI-CORONAL

FIGURE 4-4   Leiomyoma *(continued)*

4-4E   Subserous fibroid extrinsic to endometrium.

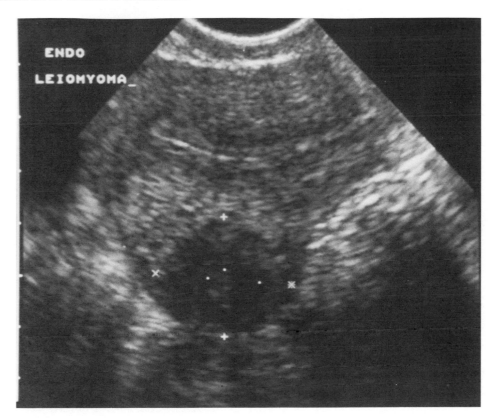

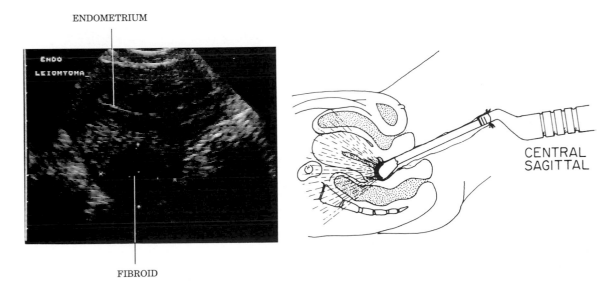

ENDOMETRIUM

FIBROID

CENTRAL
SAGITTAL

FIGURE 4-5   Endometrial Hyperplasia/Adenomyosis

4-5A Thickened endometrium in a patient with endometrial hyperplasia.

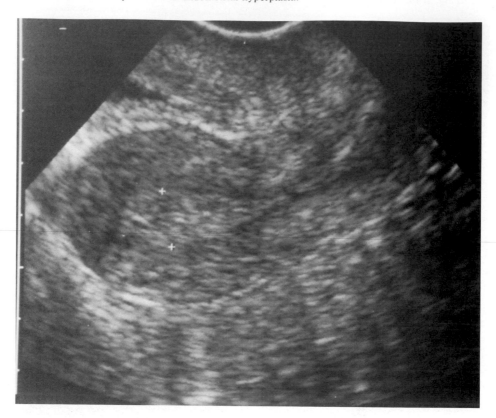

HYPERPLASTIC ENDOMETRIUM

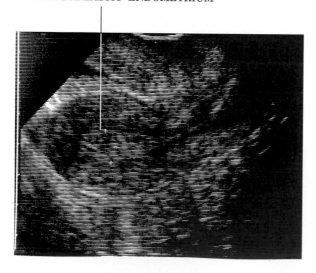

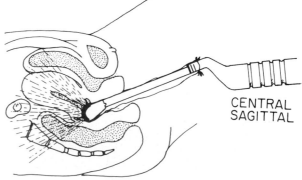

CENTRAL
SAGITTAL

FIGURE 4-5   Endometrial Hyperplasia/Adenomyosis *(continued)*

4-5B   Adenomyosis causing increased echogenicity of the myometrium.

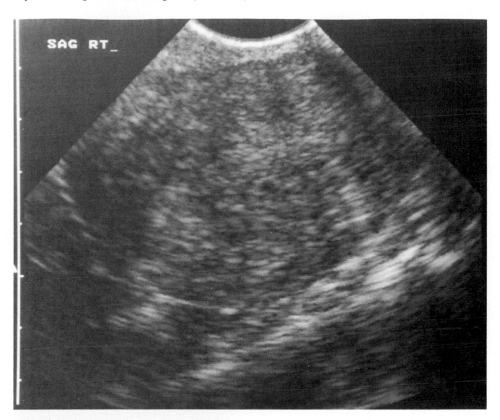

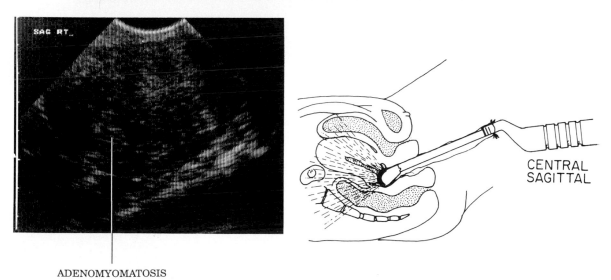

ADENOMYOMATOSIS

CENTRAL
SAGITTAL

FIGURE 4-6   TVS of Endometrial Carcinoma with Accompanying Sectioned Gross Specimen

4-6A   Diagram showing superficial (S), intermediate (I), and deep (D) myometrial invasion as determined by TVS.

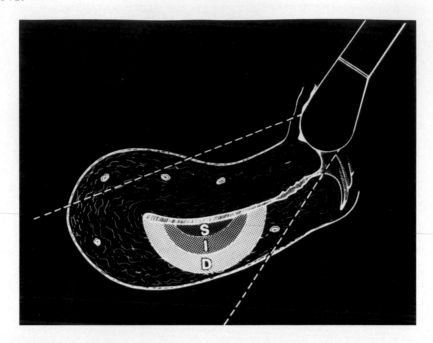

FIGURE 4-6   **TVS of Endometrial Carcinoma with Accompanying Sectioned Gross Specimen** *(continued)*

4-6B   Noninvasive tumor demonstrating distinct endometrial/myometrial interface.

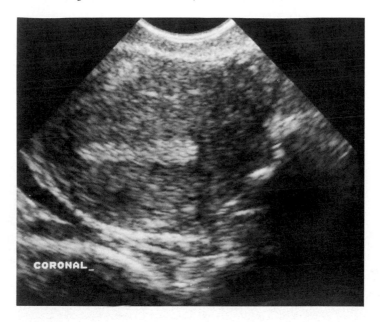

NON-INVASIVE TUMOR

UTERUS

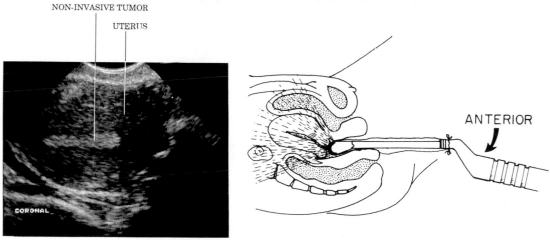

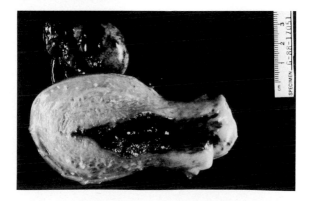

(continued)

FIGURE 4-6   **TVS of Endometrial Carcinoma with Accompanying Sectioned Gross Specimen** *(continued)*

4-6C   Superficial myometrial invasion as evidenced by focal discontinuity of subendometrial halo.

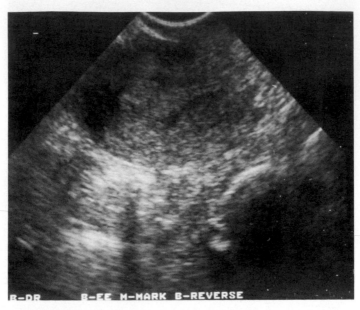

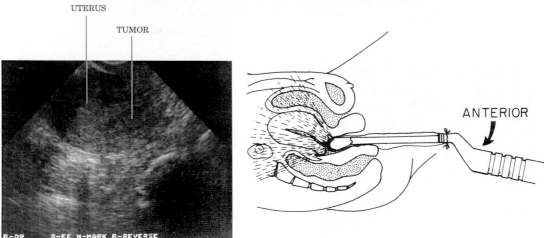

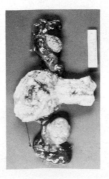

FIGURE 4-6   TVS of Endometrial Carcinoma with Accompanying Sectioned Gross Specimen *(continued)*

4-6D   Superficial myometrial invasion of bulky tumor.

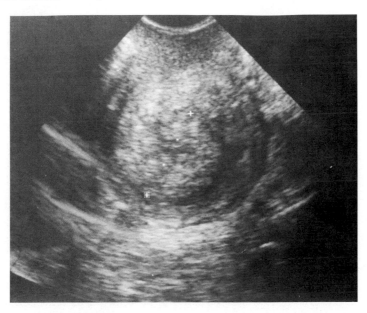

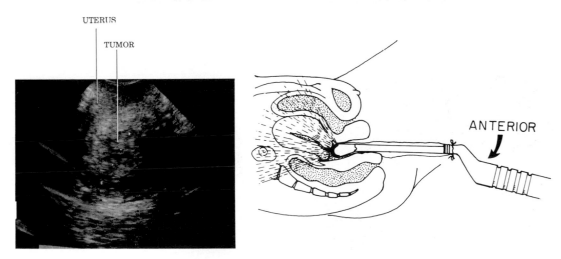

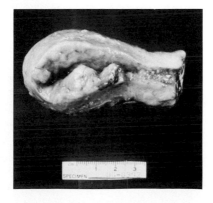

(continued)

FIGURE 4-6 **TVS of Endometrial Carcinoma with Accompanying Sectioned Gross Specimen** *(continued)*

4-6E Superficial invasion of polypoid tumor.

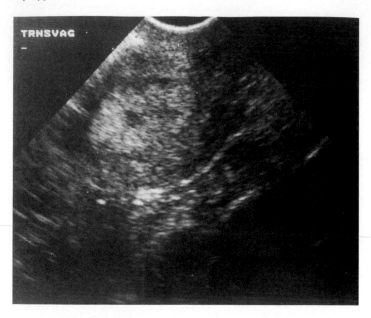

TUMOR

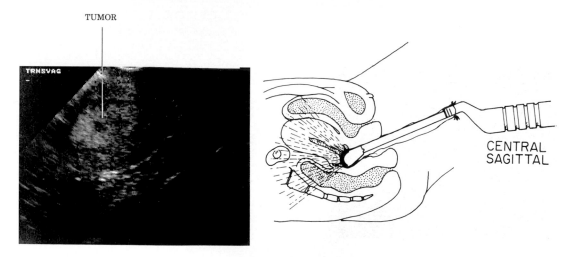

CENTRAL
SAGITTAL

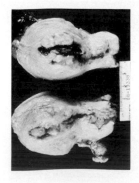

FIGURE 4-6   TVS of Endometrial Carcinoma with Accompanying Sectioned Gross Specimen *(continued)*

4-6F   Moderate myometrial invasion of hypoechoic tumor.

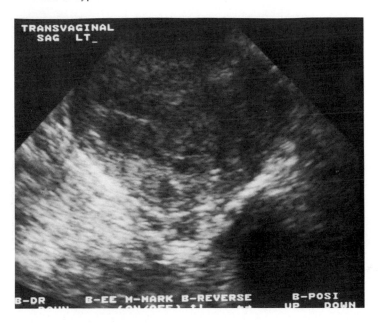

UTERUS

INVASIVE TUMOR

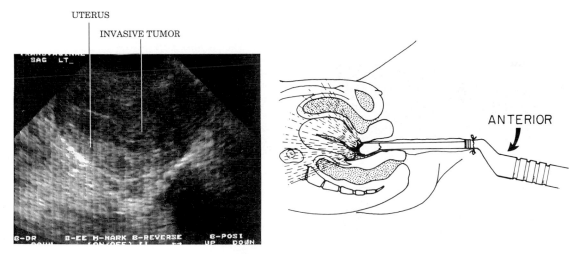

ANTERIOR

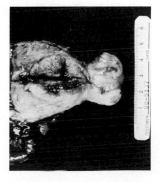

(continued)

FIGURE 4-6   TVS of Endometrial Carcinoma with Accompanying Sectioned Gross Specimen *(continued)*

4-6G   Moderately invasive polypoid tumor.

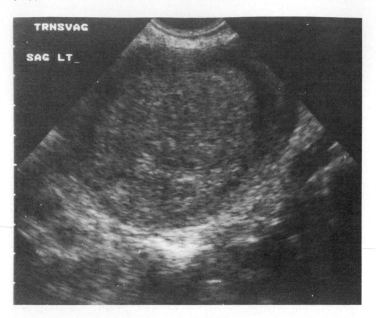

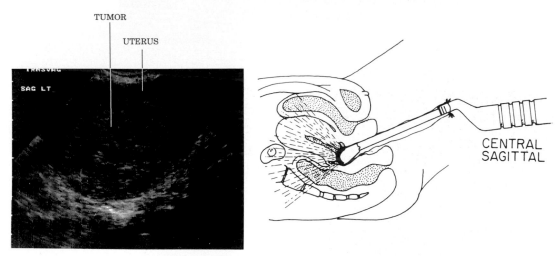

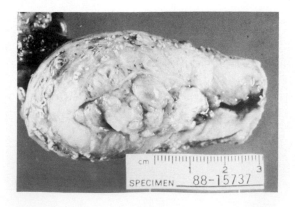

FIGURE 4-6   **TVS of Endometrial Carcinoma with Accompanying Sectioned Gross Specimen** (*continued*)

4-6H   Deep myometrial invasion within the lower uterine corpus and upper cervix. Since
it involves the cervix, this is a stage II tumor.

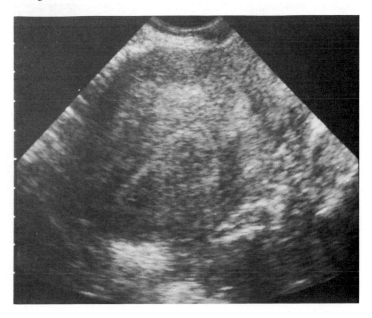

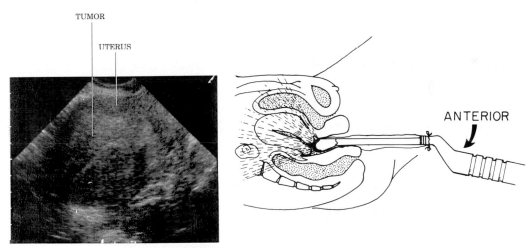

TUMOR

UTERUS

ANTERIOR

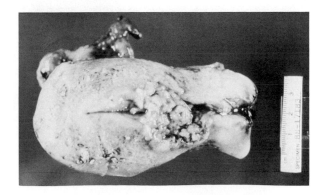

(*continued*)

FIGURE 4-6   TVS of Endometrial Carcinoma with Accompanying Sectioned Gross Specimen *(continued)*

4-6I   Deep myometrial invasion within uterine fundus.

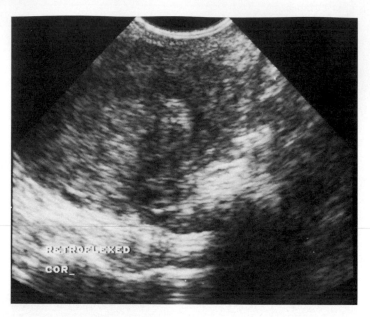

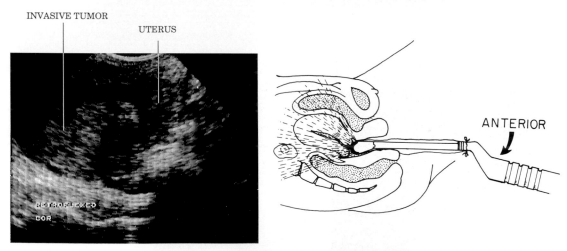

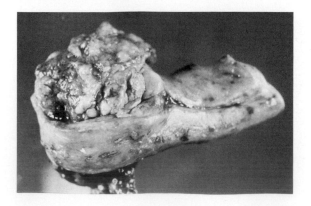

FIGURE 4-6   TVS of Endometrial Carcinoma with Accompanying Sectioned Gross Specimen *(continued)*

4-6J   Invasive polypoid tumor.

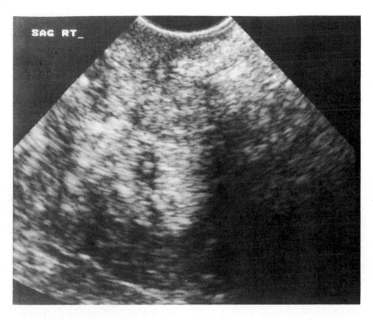

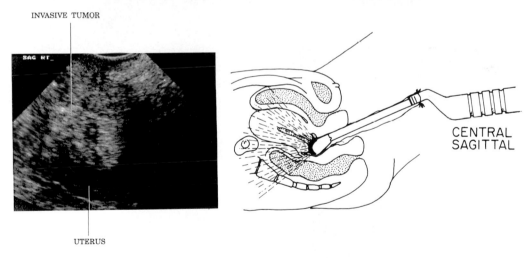

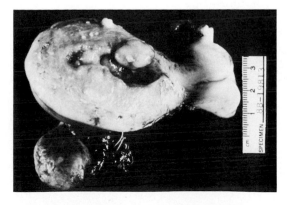

(continued)

FIGURE 4-6   TVS of Endometrial Carcinoma with Accompanying Sectioned Gross Specimen *(continued)*

4-6K   Noninvasive polypoid (papillary serous) tumor on a stalk surrounded by fluid.

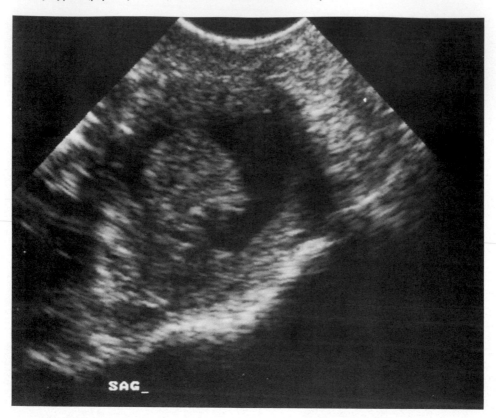

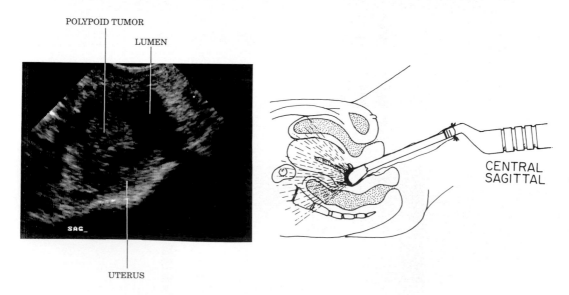

FIGURE 4-7   Presumably Invasive Endometrial Tumors that Underwent Radiation Therapy. **No surgical confirmation possible.**

4-7A   Bulky endometrial tumor extending into cervix.

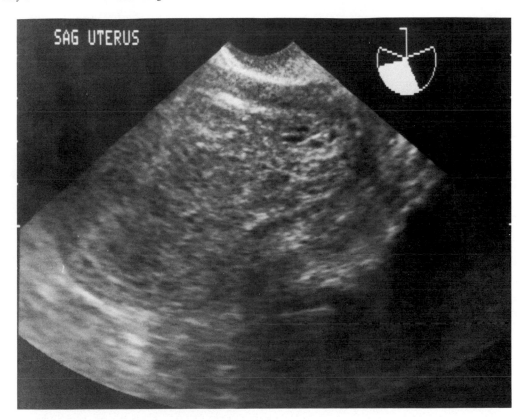

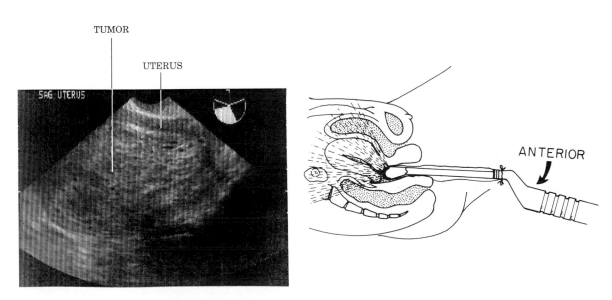

(continued)

FIGURE 4-7   **Presumably Invasive Endometrial Tumors that Underwent Radiation Therapy. No surgical confirmation possible.** *(continued)*

4-7B   Tumor extending to uterine serosa.

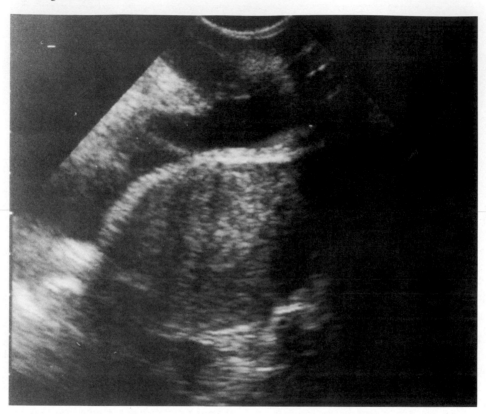

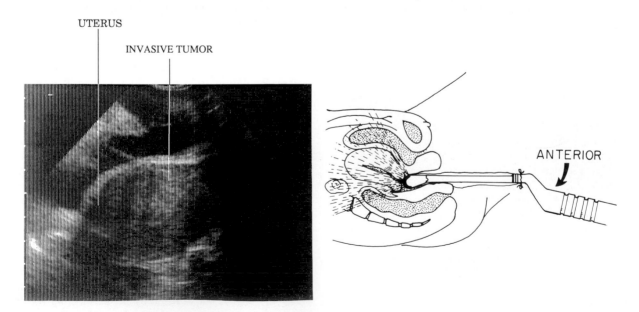

Chapter 5

Ovarian Masses

Arthur C. Fleischer, MD

Introduction

Transvaginal sonography (TVS) affords detailed delineation of the normal ovary as well as masses that are confined to the true pelvis. Masses larger than 10 cm are best evaluated using conventional transabdominal sonography, however. This chapter will emphasize both the transvaginal and transabdominal sonographic approach to evaluation of the ovarian mass. The discussion is divided into sonographic categories of ovarian masses.

Normal Ovaries

Transabdominal and transvaginal sonography can identify the ovary in the majority of premenopausal and postmenopausal women. Although it is true that in the postmenopausal patient the ovary may be difficult to identify transabdominally, in over 60% of patients, both ovaries can be identified in postmenopausal women, particularly if scanning transvaginally and using abdominal palpation (Fleischer et al, 1990; Rodriguez et al, 1988).

In premenopausal women, the normal ovary typically measures $3 \times 2 \times 1$ cm (Fig. 5-1A). It may be up to 5 cm in length in one dimension, but should remain oval in shape. Rounded ovaries typically are encountered in patients with polycystic ovarian disease. Measurement of the long, short, and anteroposterior dimension of the ovary determines ovarian volume by the prolate ellipsoid formula (length $\times$ height $\times$ width $\times$ 0.5 = volume in cm³). In premenopausal women, the normal ovary ranges from 10 to 12 cm³ in size, depending on the presence of a mature follicle, which can account for up to 2 cm or 4 cm³ of volume. In postmenopausal women, however, the normal ovary should be no larger than 8 cm³ (Campbell et al, 1982; Goswamy et al, 1988). The texture should be relatively featureless without presence of cystic or solid areas within the ovary (see Fig. 5-1B,C).

Cystic Ovarian Masses

By definition, cystic ovarian masses contain no internal echoes, a smooth wall, and demonstrate enhanced through-transmission. Cystic masses occasionally may contain low-level echoes representing blood, pus, or cellular debris. Low-level echoes may also arise from proteinaceous or mucinous material within a predominantly cystic mass. Low-level echoes may be most apparent when the ovarian mass is scanned with higher frequency transducers or by the transvaginal approach.

In premenopausal women, the most common cystic mass is the physiologic ovarian cyst (Fig. 5-2A,B). These may represent either follicular or luteal cysts, depending on when the cyst begins to form during an ovulatory cycle. Luteal cysts tend to have thicker walls than follicular cysts; both measure over 3 cm in size—greater than that expected for a mature graafian follicle. The intraovarian location of the cyst can be identified on TVS by displacement of ovarian parenchyma, forming a ''beak'' of normal ovarian tissue around the cyst (see Fig. 5-2B).

When hemorrhage occurs within the cyst, low-level echoes or thin internal septae can be identified within the ovarian mass (Fig. 5-2C). Therefore, hemorrhagic corpus lutea can mimic the appearance of a variety of ovarian masses, such as endometriomas and some epithelial tumors. Hemorrhagic corpus lutea tend to regress, however, whereas ovarian tumors and untreated endometriomas do not. Hemorrhagic cysts may precipitate ovarian torsion. Torsion can be identified using color Doppler transvaginal scanning or transabdominal scanning by the absence of arterial or venous signals from an enlarged ovary.

Other cystic masses near and around the ovary that can be identified on transabdominal or transvaginal scanning include endometriomas, paraovarian cysts, and sactosalpinges. Paraovarian cysts are separate from the ovary and are usually caused by fluid collecting within a remnant of the Gartner's duct located in the mesovarium (Fig. 5-3A). Endometriomas may have a variety of sonographic appearances, ranging from anechoic to echogenic and from loculated to septated, depending on the amount and coagulation of the internal blood components (see Fig. 5-3B). Their borders may be irregular because of the fibrosis they incite in the surrounding soft tissue. Peritoneal cysts are typically related to previous surgery. They represent fluid collections that are walled off by the serosa of the pelvic organs.

Cystic Ovarian Tumors

Ovarian cystic masses may range from 2 cm up to 30 to 40 cm in size. If they are completely anechoic and smooth-walled, they have a high probability of being benign (Goldstein et al, 1989; Andolf et al, 1986). Even in postmenopausal women in whom ovarian cancer incidence is greatest, an anechoic mass with smooth walls and good through-transmission has a greater than 95% incidence of being benign (Goldstein et al, 1989; Andolf and Jörgensen, 1989). If there is any question as to the possibility of malignancy, a CA-125 assay may be performed to detect the ovarian tumor in a patient with a completely cystic mass.

Ovarian epithelial tumors have a variety of internal consistencies ranging from septated, papillary excrescences, or irregular solid components. Mucinous tumors tend to have thin internal septae and may have areas of echogenic material within them that arise from mucin (Fig. 5-4A). Serous cystadenomas tend to be hypoechoic and unilocular, whereas epithelial carcinomas may demonstrate internal papillary excrescences (see Fig. 5-4B,C). Echogenic internal material that is mobile may be the result of either hemorrhage, cellular debris, or, in dermoid cysts, sebum that layers above the serous content of the dermoid cyst.

Complex Ovarian Masses

Complex ovarian masses represent lesions that contain both cystic and solid components. The most common of these is the dermoid cyst, although ovarian epithelial tumors, when large, frequently have a complex appearance.

Dermoid cysts demonstrate a variety of sonographic appearances, ranging from anechoic to echogenic. Anechoic dermoid cysts tend to arise from neuroectoderm and are encountered in young girls, whereas solid dermoid cysts tend to represent teratomas, some of which can be malignant, particularly in adolescents. The most common appearance of a dermoid cyst is a mass that has cystic and solid components (Fig. 5-5A to D). The solid areas represent hair follicles and solid tissue

combined with echogenic foci that represent calcified elements within the dermoid cysts. Some dermoid cysts contain sebum, a buttery material that tends to layer anteriorly within dermoid cysts because of its low specific gravity (see Fig. 5-5E).

Complex ovarian masses most frequently arise from masses containing hemorrhage such as the hemorrhagic corpus luteum. Endometriomas may also demonstrate this appearance, as do some types of hemorrhagic ovarian masses in patients with bleeding disorders (Fig. 5-6A to D).

Solid Ovarian Tumors

Compared with cystic ovarian tumors, solid ones are relatively uncommon (Fig. 5-7A,B). Solid ovarian tumors typically arise from either primary or secondary adenocarcinoma of the ovary or the less differentiated ovarian tumors. Solid ovarian tumors may be differentiated from pedunculated fibroids by the transvaginal route. When pelvic or abdominal pressure is applied to the mass, one should be able to separate a uterine from an ovarian lesion. Metastases to the ovary are not uncommon and usually present as solid ovarian masses.

Early Detection of Ovarian Carcinoma

Several reports on the possible use of transabdominal or transvaginal sonography in the screening and early detection of patients with ovarian carcinoma have been encouraging. Campbell's series of over 5000 women has demonstrated the efficacy of such a program that uses transabdominal sonography (Campbell, et al, 1989). Five patients with primary ovarian cancer were found, all with stage I tumors. Higgins' study involving 500 patients also demonstrated the efficacy of TVS in the early detection of ovarian tumors (Higgins et al, 1989). Jacobs' study and Finkler's work have demonstrated the efficacy of using both transabdominal sonography and CA-125 assay as early detection programs (Jacobs et al, 1988; Finkler et al, 1988).

Although ovarian carcinoma occurs in 1 of 70 women in the United States, one can argue that its detection in its early stages is worthwhile because most ovarian tumors are discovered in later stages if left to clinical discovery. Our study has shown that TVS has significant negative predictive value in that if an ovarian mass is not shown, the patient most likely does not have an ovarian tumor (Fig. 5-8A to F) (Fleischer et al, 1990).

It is possible that the addition of transvaginal color Doppler sonography may help detect ovarian lesions, particularly those that incite significant neovascularization (Fleischer et al, 1990; Bourne et al, 1989). Considering the large number of women that need to be screened, the best hope for early detection seems to lie in the combination of sensitive serum assay and sonography.

Paraovarian Masses

Some paraovarian masses may appear to arise from the ovaries, especially when the compressed rim of ovarian tumor that usually surrounds an intraovarian mass cannot be detected (Fig. 5-9). These masses normally represent endometriosis that is attached to the ovarian serosa or paraovarian masses that arise from the mesoovarium.

Summary

This chapter has outlined the sonographic appearances of most ovarian tumors using both transabdominal and transvaginal sonography. The use of transabdominal and transvaginal sonography for the early detection of ovarian carcinoma seems promising and should be pursued by several institutions in clinical trials.

References

Andolf E, Svalenius E, Astedt B. Ultrasonography for early detection of ovarian carcinoma. *Br J Obstet Gynaecol* 1986;93:1286–1289.

Andolf E, Jörgensen C. Cystic lesions in elderly women, diagnosed by ultrasound. *Br J Obstet Gynaecol* 1989; 96:1076–1079.

Bourne T, Campbell S, Steer C, Whitehead MI, Collins WP. Transvaginal colour flow imaging: a possible new screening technique for ovarian cancer. *Br Med J* 1989;299:1367–1370.

Campbell S, Bhan V, Royston P, Whitehead MI, Collins WP. Transabdominal ultrasound screening for early ovarian cancer. *Br Med J* 1989;299:1363–1367.

Campbell S, Goessens L, Goswamy R, Whitehead MI. Real-time ultrasonography for the determination of ovarian morphology and volume: a possible early screening test for ovarian cancer. *Lancet* 1982;1:425–426.

Finkler NJ, Benacerraf B, Wojciechowski C, Lavin PT, Knapp RC. Comparison of serum CA 125, clinical impression, and ultrasound in the preoperative evaluation of ovarian masses. *Obstet Gynecol* 1988;72:659.

Fleischer AC, Kepple DM, Rao BK, Jeanty P. Transvaginal color Doppler sonography: preliminary experience. *Dynamic Cardiovasc Imaging* 1990;3:52–55.

Fleischer AC, Gordon A, McKee M, et al. Transvaginal sonography of postmenopausal ovaries with pathologic correlation. *J Ultrasound Med* 1990;9:637–640.

Goldstein SR, Subramanyam B, Snyder JR, Beller U, Raghavendra BN, Beckman EM. The postmenopausal cystic adnexal mass: the potential role of ultrasound in conservative management. *Obstet Gynecol* 1989;74:8.

Goswamy RK, Campbell S, Royston JP, et al. Ovarian size in postmenopausal women. *Br J Obstet Gynaecol* 1988; 95:795–801.

Higgins RV, van Nagell JR Jr, Donaldson ES, et al. Transvaginal sonography as a screening method for ovarian cancer. *Gynecol Oncol* 1989;34:402–406.

Jacobs I, Stabile I, Bridges J, et al. Multimodal approach to screening for ovarian cancer. *Lancet* 1988;1:268–271.

Rodriguez MH, Platt LD, Medearis AL, Lacarra M, Lobo RA. The use of transvaginal sonography for evaluation of postmenopausal ovarian size and morphology. *Am J Obstet Gynecol* 1988;159:810–814.

FIGURE 5-1   Normal Ovaries

5-1A   Transvaginal sonogram of a postmenopausal woman demonstrating normal right ovary (between cursors).

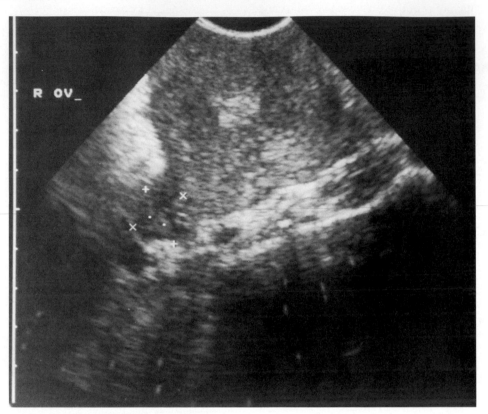

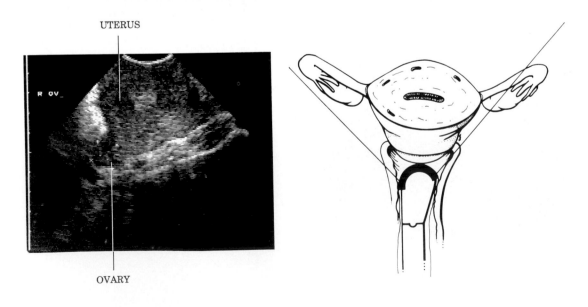

UTERUS

OVARY

FIGURE 5-1   Normal Ovaries *(continued)*

5-1B   Fresh corpus luteum within left ovary.

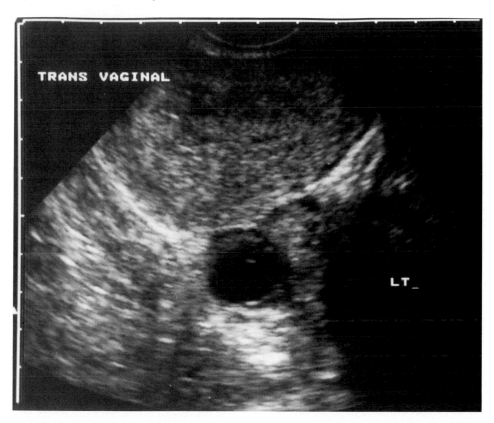

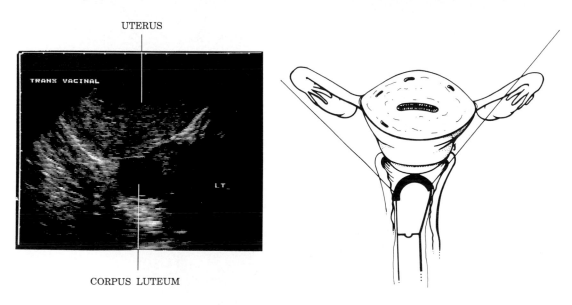

UTERUS

CORPUS LUTEUM

(continued)

FIGURE 5-1   Normal Ovaries (*continued*)

5-1C   Normal right ovary in perimenopausal woman. The resected uterus and ovaries show that the right ovary was twice the size of the left.

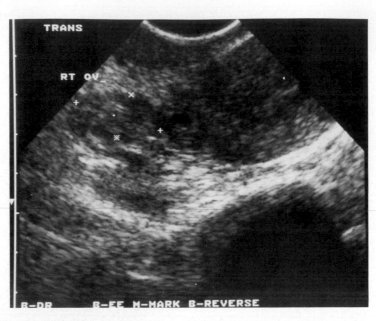

OVARY

UTERUS

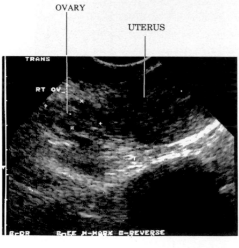

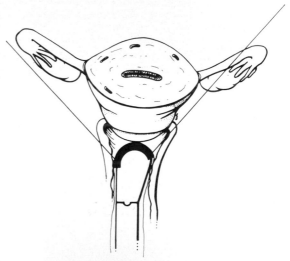

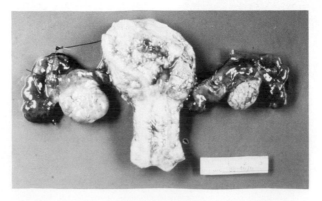

FIGURE 5-2   Cystic Masses

5-2A   Transabdominal sonogram demonstrating the appearance of a nonspecific right adnexal cystic mass (between cursors).

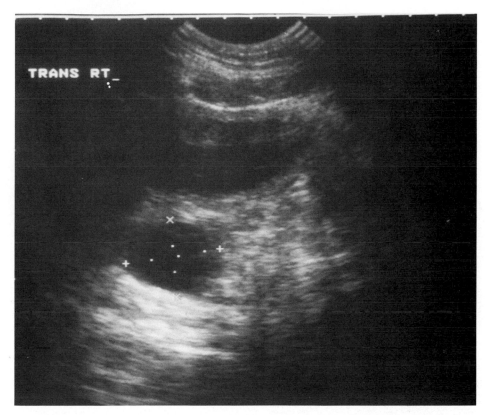

(continued)

FIGURE 5-2   Cystic Masses *(continued)*

5-2B   Transvaginal sonogram of patient in *A* demonstrating intraovarian cyst (between cursors). Note the displacement of normal ovarian tissue surrounding the cyst.

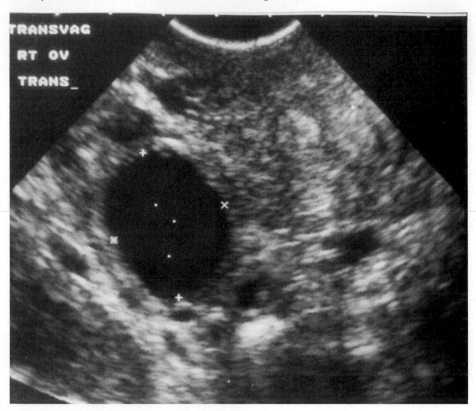

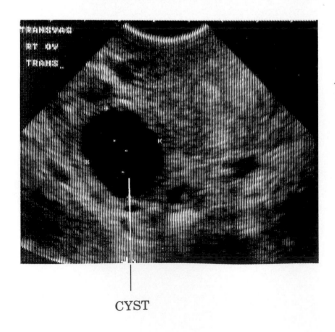

CYST

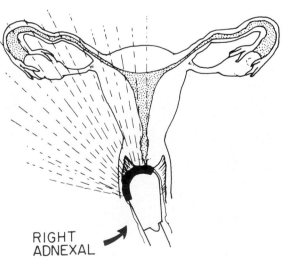

RIGHT
ADNEXAL

FIGURE 5-2 Cystic Masses *(continued)*

5-2C Transvaginal sonogram of hemorrhagic corpus luteum demonstrating low-level
internal echoes.

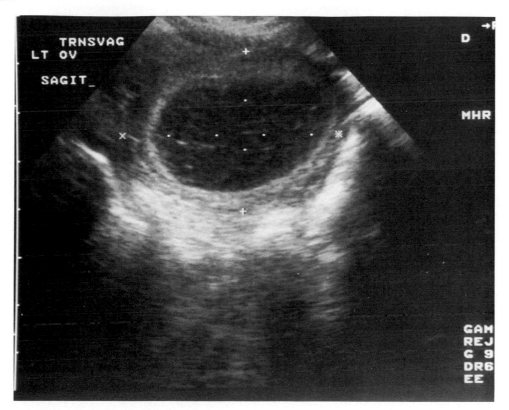

HEMORRHAGIC CORPUS LUTEUM CYST

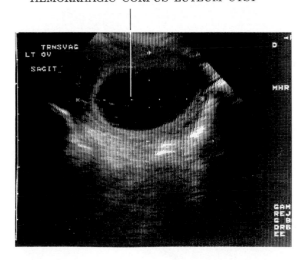

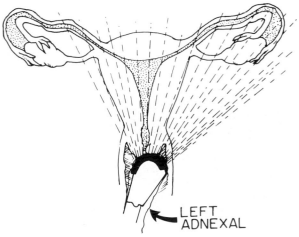

LEFT
ADNEXAL

FIGURE 5-3   Extraovarian Adnexal Masses

5-3A   Transvaginal sonogram of paraovarian cyst adjacent to left ovary.

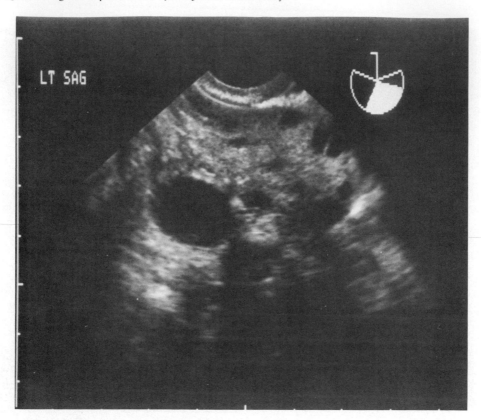

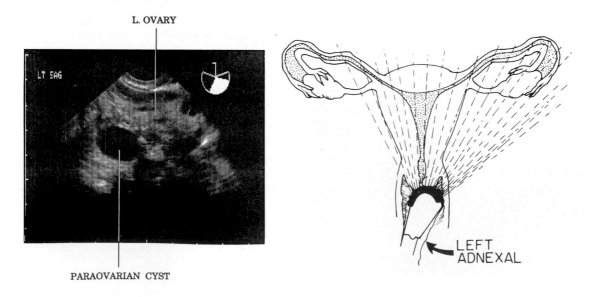

FIGURE 5-3   Extraovarian Adnexal Masses *(continued)*

5-3B   Transvaginal sonogram of endometrioma adjacent to right ovary containing echogenic organized blood.

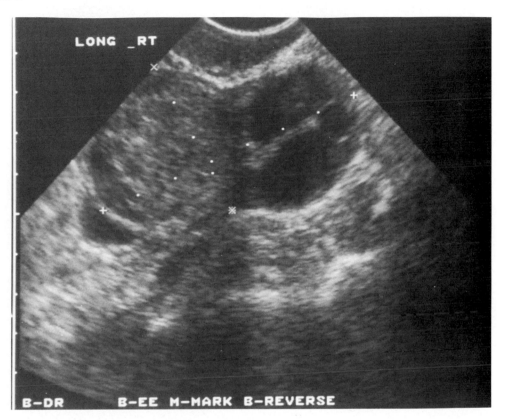

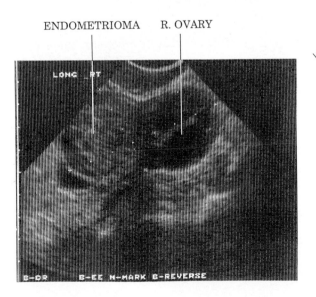

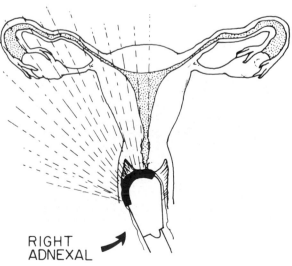

FIGURE 5-4   Predominately Cystic Ovarian Tumors

5-4A   Transvaginal sonogram showing a cystic mass in right ovary with a slightly irregular wall.

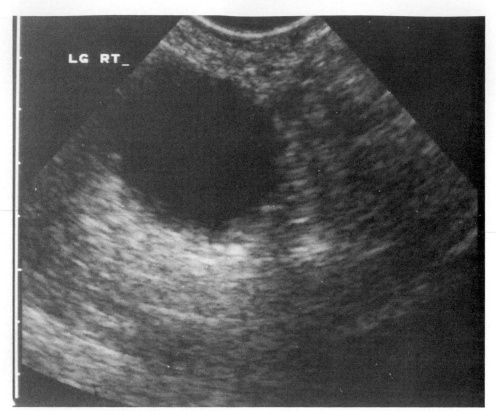

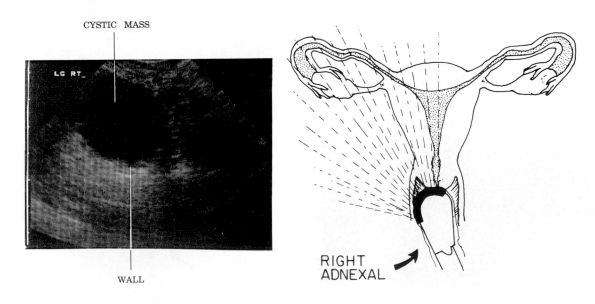

FIGURE 5-4   **Predominately Cystic Ovarian Tumors** *(continued)*

5-4B   Same patient as *A* demonstrating a 3-cm septated mass in left ovary. This patient had bilateral serous cystadenomas.

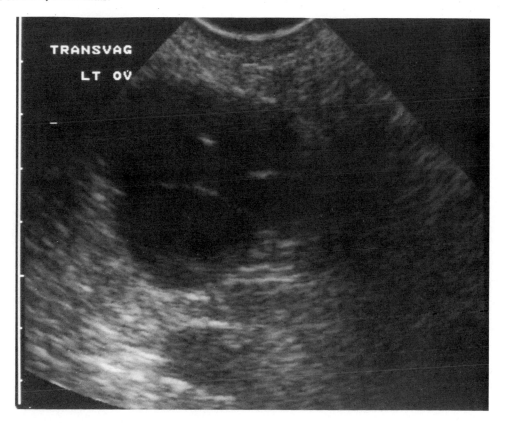

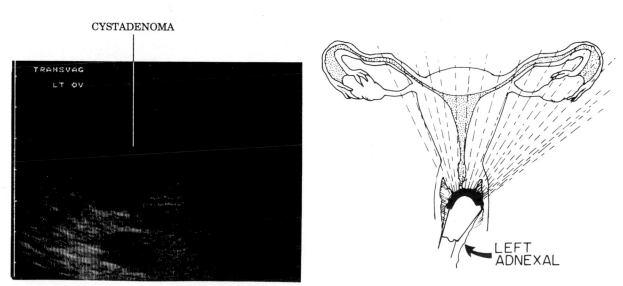

(continued)

FIGURE 5-4   **Predominately Cystic Ovarian Tumors** *(continued)*

5-4C   Transvaginal sonogram demonstrating bilateral cystic masses containing septae and solid components representing bilateral mucinous cystadenomas.

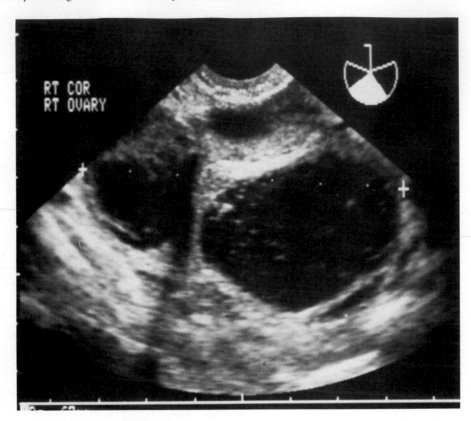

OVARIAN CYSTADENOMAS

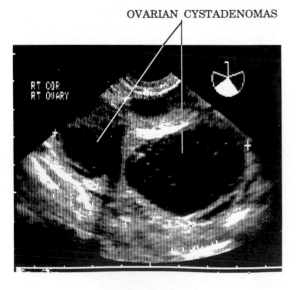

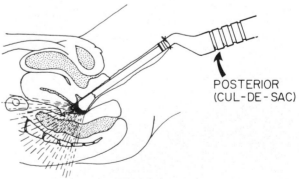

POSTERIOR
(CUL-DE-SAC)

FIGURE 5-4   **Predominately Cystic Ovarian Tumors** *(continued)*

5-4D   Cystic mass containing papillary excresences. This was a metastasis from a gastrointestinal tract tumor.

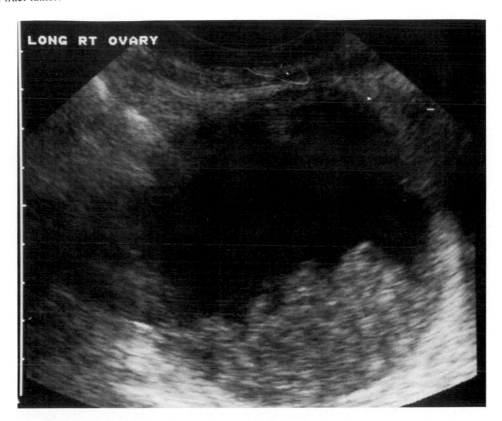

PAPILLARY   EXCRESENCES

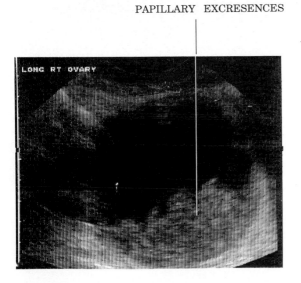

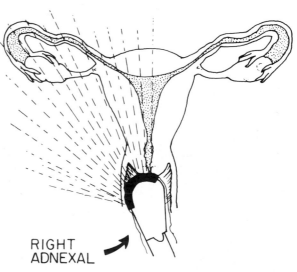

FIGURE 5-5   Dermoid Cyst

5-5A   Transabdominal sonogram demonstrating cystic mass superior to right ovary. Right ovary contains an echogenic focus.

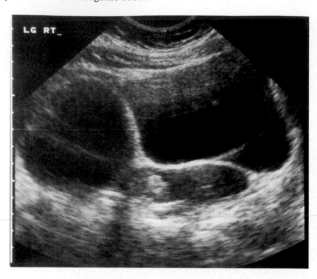

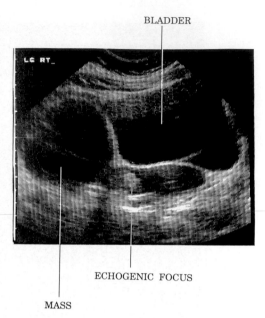

5-5B   Transabdominal sonogram of same patient in *A* demonstrating cystic mass in left adnexa with echogenic internal component.

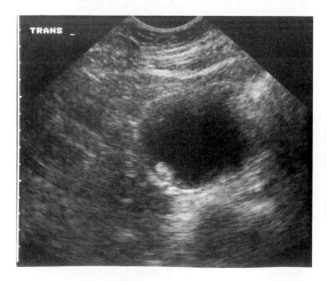

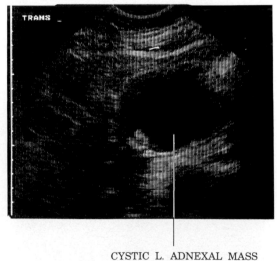

FIGURE 5-5   Dermoid Cyst *(continued)*

5-5C   Transvaginal sonogram of same patient as *B* showing left adnexal mass with echogenic mobile material. Patient had bilateral dermoid cysts.

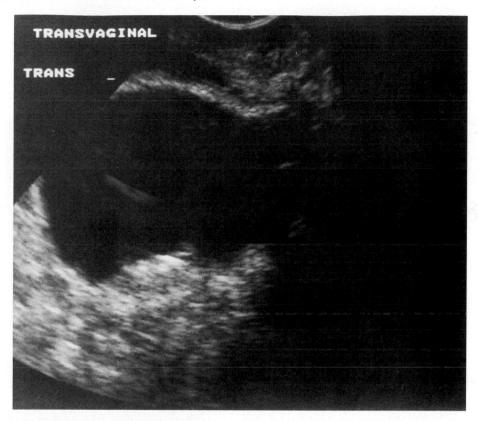

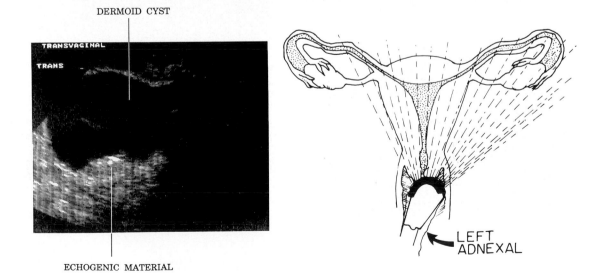

DERMOID CYST

ECHOGENIC MATERIAL

LEFT ADNEXAL

(continued)

FIGURE 5-5   Dermoid Cyst *(continued)*

5-5D   Transvaginal sonogram of dermoid cyst with a layer of sebum.

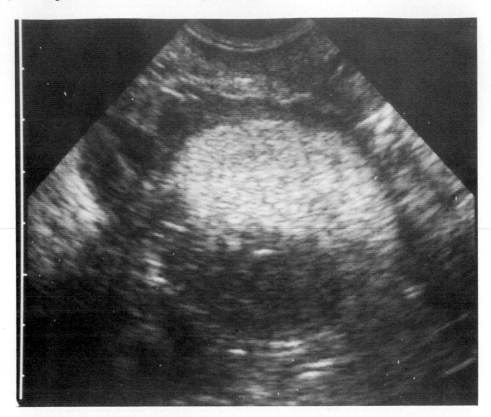

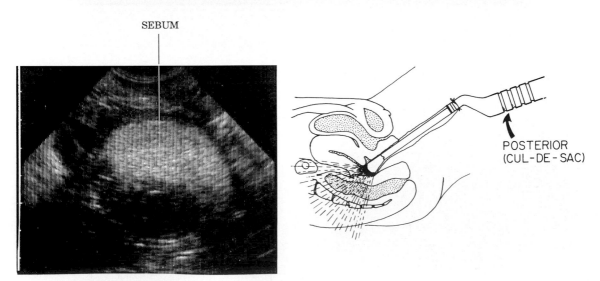

SEBUM

POSTERIOR
(CUL-DE-SAC)

FIGURE 5-5   **Dermoid Cyst** *(continued)*

5-5E   Dermoid containing echogenic teeth.

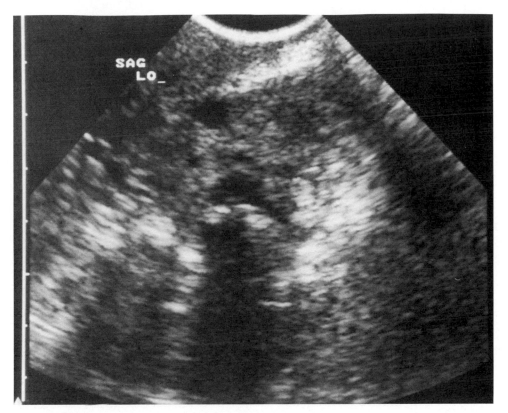

CALCIFICATIONS

LEFT
ADNEXAL

(continued)

FIGURE 5-5   Dermoid Cyst *(continued)*

5-5F Nonspecific echogenic area found to represent a dermoid cyst at surgery.

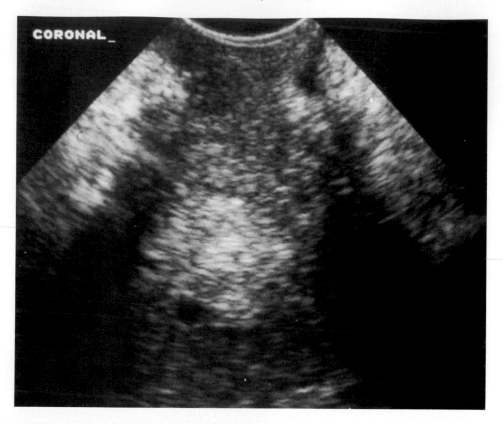

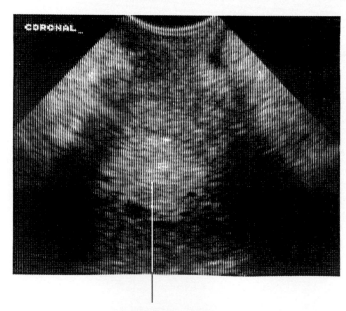

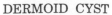

DERMOID CYST

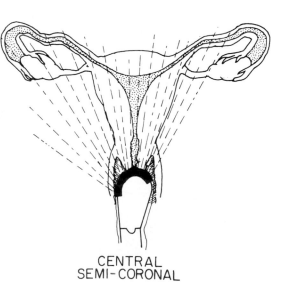

CENTRAL
SEMI-CORONAL

FIGURE 5-5 Dermoid Cyst *(continued)*

5-5G Opened specimen of *F* showing abundant hair.

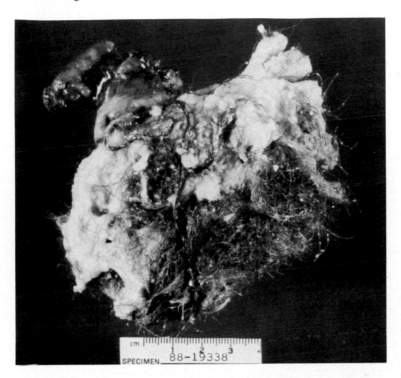

FIGURE 5-6   Complex Ovarian Masses

5-6A   Transvaginal sonogram of a 10-cm complex mass containing internal echoes and septae, representing a hemorrhagic corpus luteum cyst.

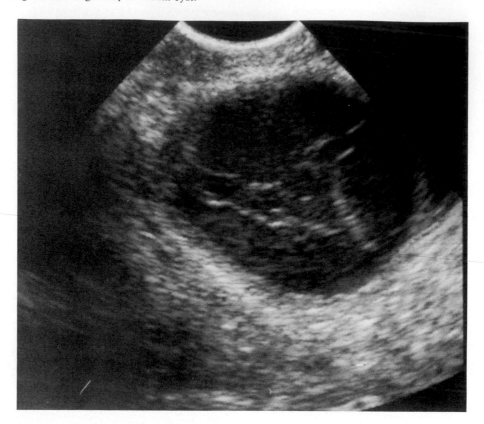

HEMORRHAGIC CORPUS LUTEUM CYST

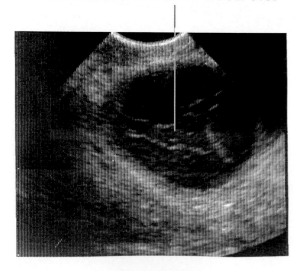

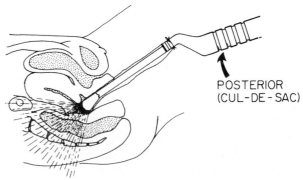

POSTERIOR
(CUL-DE-SAC)

FIGURE 5-6   Complex Ovarian Masses *(continued)*

5-6B   Transvaginal sonogram showing complex mass with an irregular solid wall, representing an ovarian metastasis

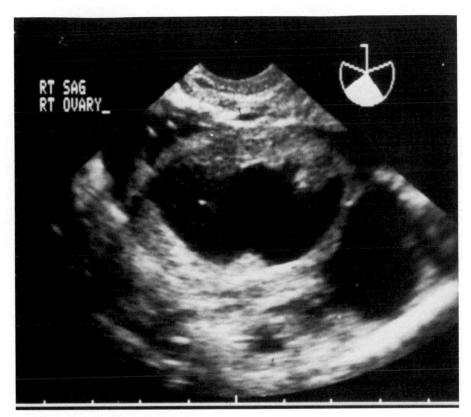

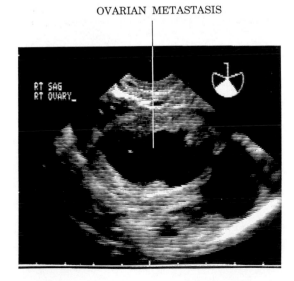

OVARIAN METASTASIS

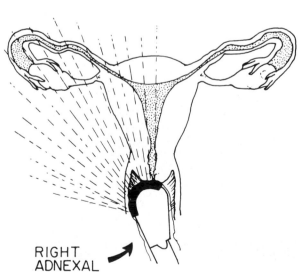

RIGHT
ADNEXAL

(continued)

FIGURE 5-6   Complex Ovarian Masses *(continued)*

5-6C   Enlarged ovary containing a tubo-ovarian abscess.

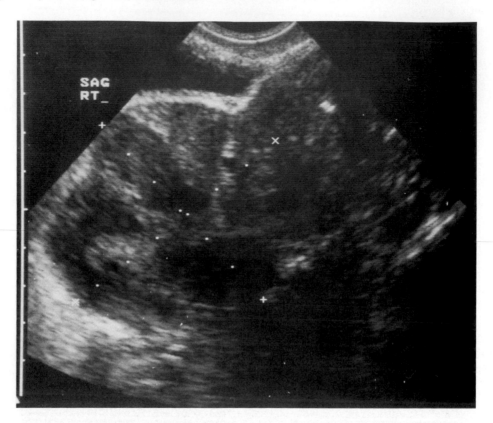

TUBO- OVARIAN ABSCESS

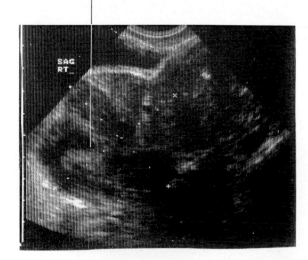

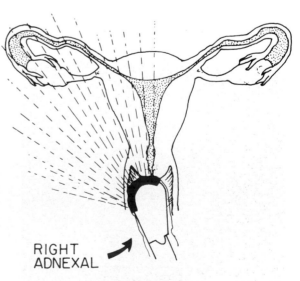

RIGHT
ADNEXAL

FIGURE 5-6   Complex Ovarian Masses *(continued)*

5-6D   Large solid mass representing a hemorrhagic ovarian cyst compressing the remaining normal portion of the left ovary.

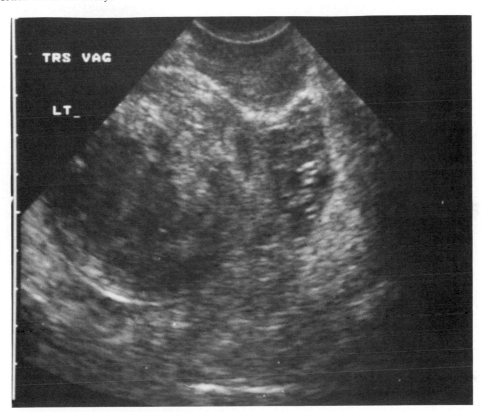

HEMORRHAGIC OVARIAN CYST

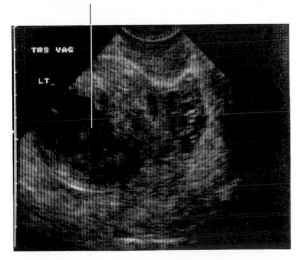

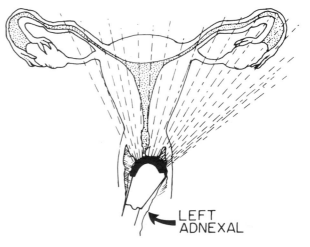

FIGURE 5-7   Solid Ovarian Masses

5-7A   Transabdominal sonogram showing hypoechoic mass in left adnexa (between cursors).

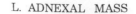

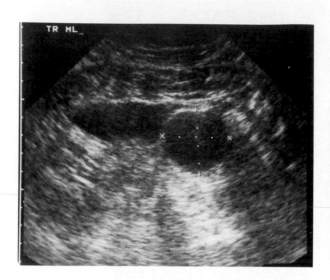
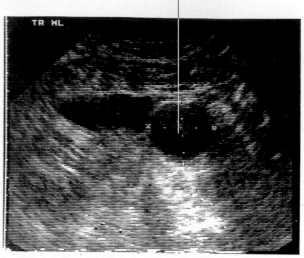

FIGURE 5-7   Solid Ovarian Masses *(continued)*

5-7B   Transvaginal sonogram of patient in *A* showing solid ovarian mass adjacent to cystic one. A torsed endometrioma was identified, as was a physiologic ovarian cyst in the left ovary.

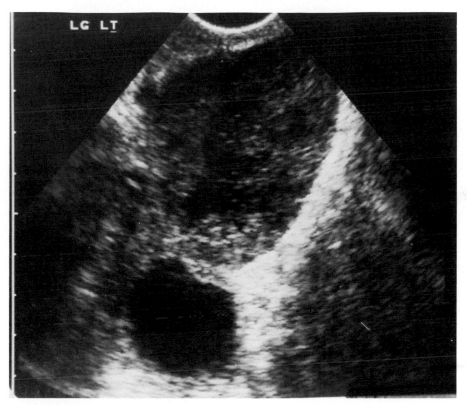

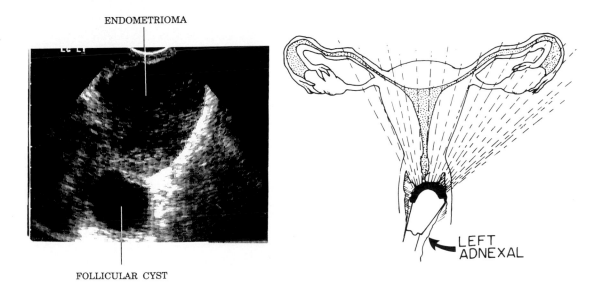

ENDOMETRIOMA

FOLLICULAR CYST

LEFT ADNEXAL

(continued)

FIGURE 5-7   Solid Ovarian Masses *(continued)*

5-7C   Gross specimen of *A* and *B* showing torsed endometrioma within gangrenous ovary.

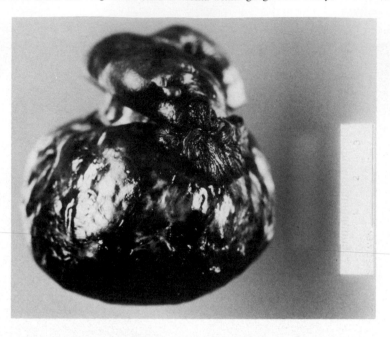

FIGURE 5-7 **Solid Ovarian Masses** *(continued)*

5-7D   Enlarged right ovary with hemorrhagic area.

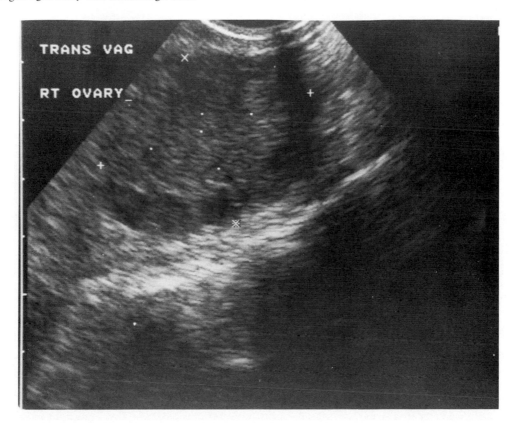

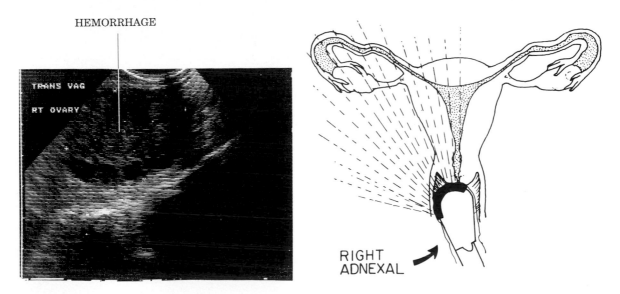

(continued)

FIGURE 5-7   Solid Ovarian Masses (*continued*)

5-7E   Same patient as in *D*. Loculated cul-de-sac fluid is seen. A torsed right ovary was found at surgery.

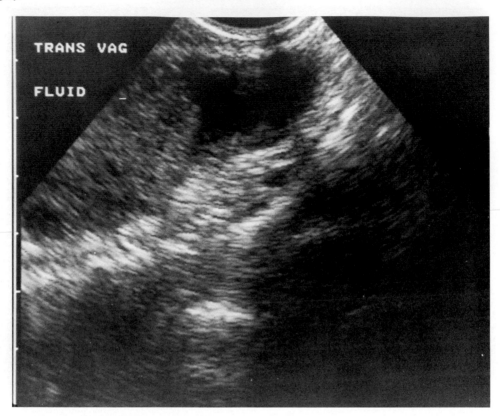

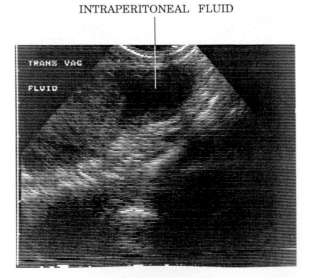

INTRAPERITONEAL FLUID

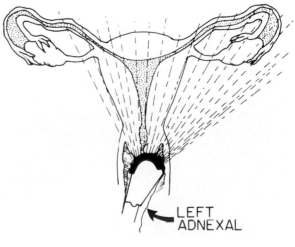

LEFT ADNEXAL

FIGURE 5-8 Small (<5 cm) Ovarian Lesions in Postmenopausal Women with Nonpalpable Ovaries

5-8A Transvaginal sonogram of right ovary showing small solid area (between cursors).

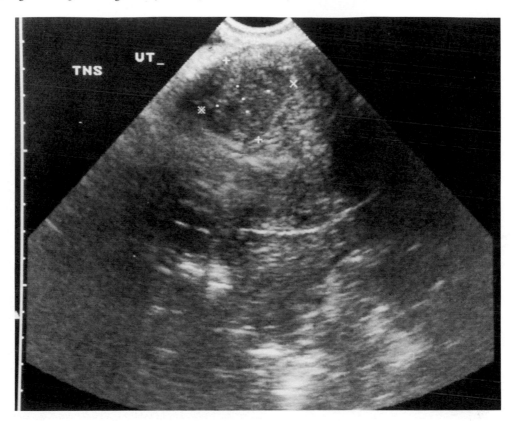

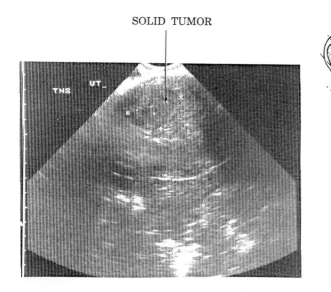

SOLID TUMOR

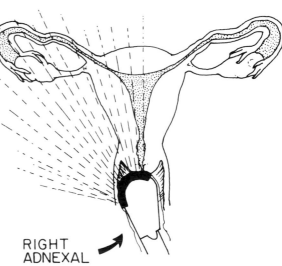

RIGHT ADNEXAL

(continued)

FIGURE 5-8   Small (<5 cm) Ovarian Lesions in Postmenopausal Women with Nonpalpable Ovaries *(continued)*

5-8B   Sectioned specimen of *A* showing an 18-mm Sertoli cell tumor adjacent to a simple cyst.

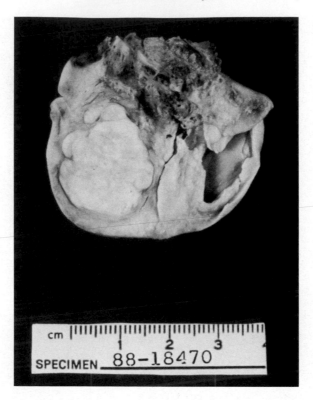

FIGURE 5-8   Small (<5 cm) Ovarian Lesions in Postmenopausal Women with Nonpalpable Ovaries *(continued)*

5-8C   Transvaginal sonogram of right ovary with cystic area (between cursors).

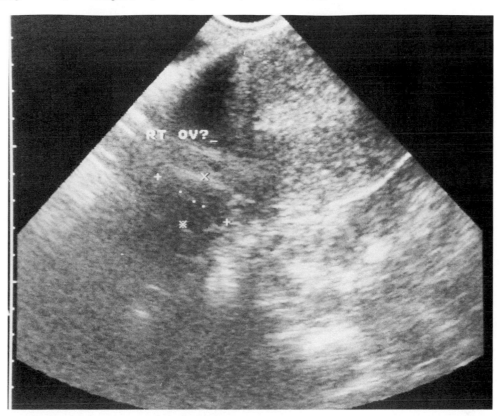

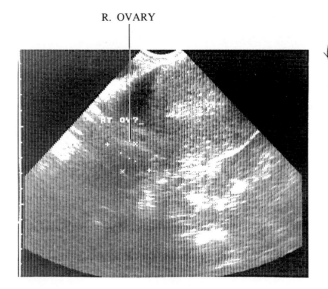

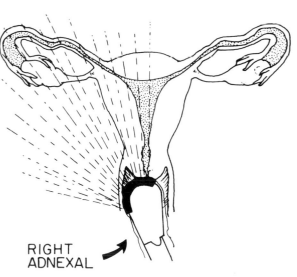

(continued)

FIGURE 5-8   Small (<5 cm) Ovarian Lesions in Postmenopausal Women with Nonpalpable Ovaries *(continued)*

5-8D   Resected ovary in *C* showing a 2-cm cystadenoma projecting from the right ovary.

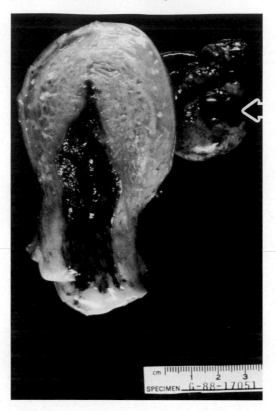

FIGURE 5-8 Small (<5 cm) Ovarian Lesions in Postmenopausal Women with Nonpalpable Ovaries *(continued)*

5-8E Transvaginal sonogram of left ovary showing complex mass with cystic and solid components.

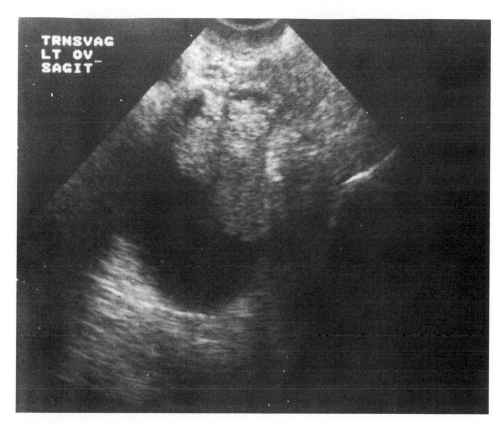

ENDOMETROID TUMOR

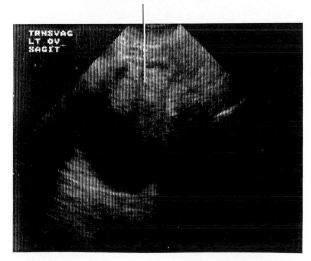

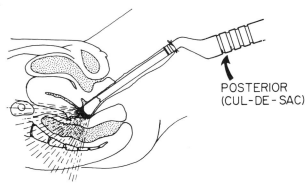

POSTERIOR (CUL-DE-SAC)

(continued)

FIGURE 5-8   Small (<5 cm) Ovarian Lesions in Postmenopausal Women with Nonpalpable Ovaries *(continued)*

5-8F   Sectioned specimen showing endometriod tumor containing solid areas.

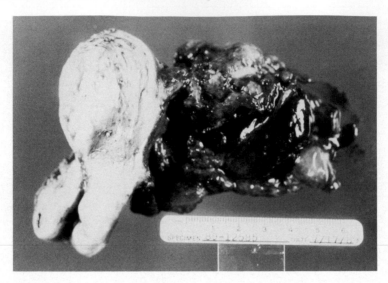

FIGURE 5-9   Paraovarian and Tubal Lesions

5-9A   Cystic area adjacent to left ovary.

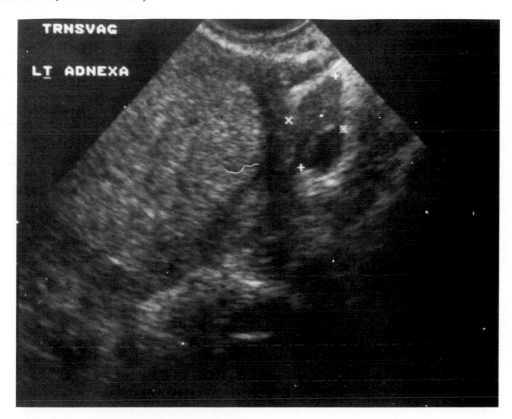

CYSTIC MASS

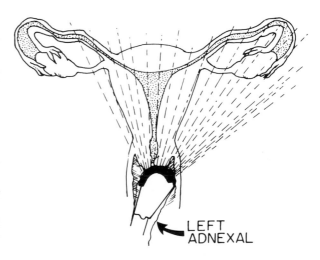

LEFT ADNEXAL

(continued)

FIGURE 5-9   Paraovarian and Tubal Lesions *(continued)*

5-9B   Same as in *A*. The cystic structure appears as a tubular mass when imaged in its long axis.

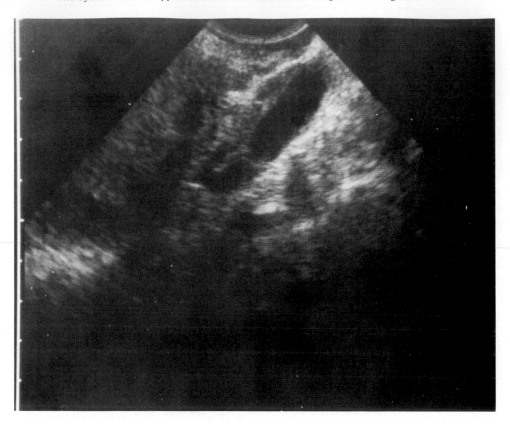

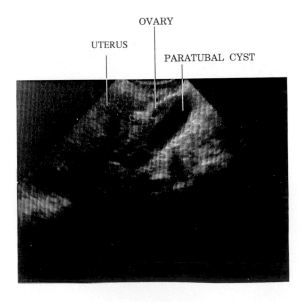

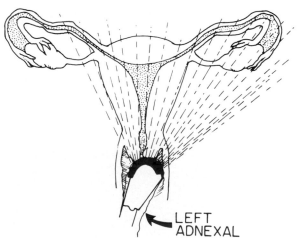

FIGURE 5-9   Paraovarian and Tubal Lesions *(continued)*

5-9C   Gross specimen of *A* and *B* showing opened paraovarian cyst adjacent to normal atrophic left ovary (curved arrow).

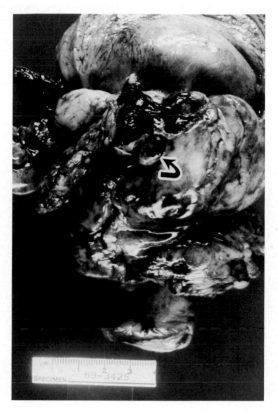

(continued)

FIGURE 5-9   Paraovarian and Tubal Lesions *(continued)*

5-9D   Fusiform solid mass adjacent to fibroid uterus.

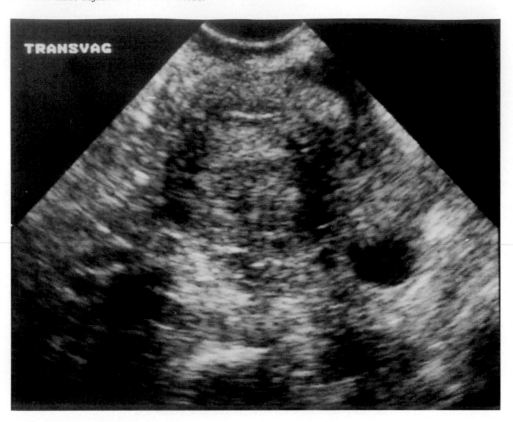

UTERUS

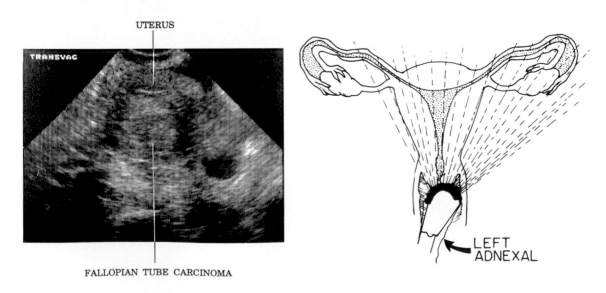

FALLOPIAN TUBE CARCINOMA

LEFT ADNEXAL

FIGURE 5-9 **Paraovarian and Tubal Lesions** *(continued)*

5-9E Resected specimen showing fallopian tube carcinoma.

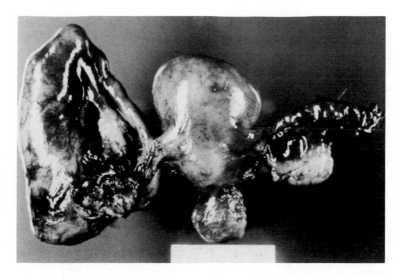

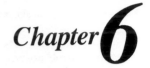

Chapter 6

Infertility

Arthur C. Fleischer, MD
Donna M. Kepple, RDMS

Introduction

The increased use and availability of transvaginal transducer-probes have had a major impact on the management and treatment of patients with gynecologic infertility (Winfield et al, 1990). Transvaginal sonography (TVS) has its greatest clinical impact in precise monitoring of follicular development, guided follicular or cyst aspiration, and guided transcervical cannulization of the fallopian tube. Other applications of TVS include evaluation of the adequacy of endometrial development and evaluation of vascular perfusion of the ovary and uterus with duplex and/or color Doppler sonography.

Follicular Monitoring

As stated previously, TVS has a vital role in depicting follicular development in patients treated for infertility that can be traced to disorders of ovulation (Fleischer et al, 1983). Although the maturity of the oocyte is only indirectly inferred by the size of the follicle, the sonographic information can be coupled with serum estradiol values to provide an accurate assessment of the presence or absence and number of mature follicles (Ritchie, 1986; Tarlatizis et al, 1984). The anatomic information obtained with TVS concerning the size and development of maturing follicles and corpora lutea can be used to distinguish physiologic from insufficient or abnormal cycles (McArdle et al, 1983; Geisthovel et al, 1983). For example, the maximal follicle size in insufficient cycles has been reported to be significantly less than in normal ones, and the absence of a corpus luteum was found more often in insufficient (luteal phase inadequate) cycles (Geisthovel et al, 1983). In addition, the undesirable development of multiple immature follicles rather than development of a single dominant follicle can be seen in patients with polycystic ovaries (Hann et al, 1984).

Although its actual contribution to infertility is controversial, some infertility specialists describe an abnormality in ovulation called luteinized unruptured follicle (LUF) syndrome as a cause of unexplained infertility (Liukkonen et al, 1984). In LUF there is failure of extrusion of the oocyte, which remains trapped within the follicle. The presence of this abnormality can be confirmed only by laparoscopic observation of the absence of a stigma (healed rent where ovulation occurred) in the ovarian capsule. Since this may not be present as little as 2 hours after ovulation, the presence of this syndrome is difficult to confirm. With TVS, one can observe failure of the follicle to deflate and the absence of intraperitoneal fluid associated with ovulation. This syndrome may be more common in women with endometriosis and may not be present in consecutive cycles (Geisthovel et al, 1983; Liukkonen et al, 1984).

Some have also reported on the "empty follicle syndrome," where a cumulus cannot be identified within the follicle (Hilgers, 1989). Although it is tempting to use TVS to assess whether or not an oocyte is present, it is believed that documentation of the cumulus does not have sufficient reliability at present to confidently diagnose this entity.

SPONTANEOUS OVULATION

At the time of birth, the female neonate has approximately 2,000,000 primary oocytes within each ovary. When menarche begins, approximately 200,000 remain per ovary. During the childbearing years, approximately 200 oocytes will be ovulated. This indicates that approximately 99.9% of primary oocytes become atretic or do not develop at all.

Maturation of the oocyte and follicle is responsive primarily to changes in follicle stimulating hormone (FSH), luteinizing hormone (LH), and circulating levels of estrogen (E_2). With the elaboration and release of

FSH in the late secretory phase, there is development of several follicles. Only one and sometimes two become dominant, however; the remainder become atretic follicles. The follicle begins its maturation process several months before actual ovulation of the oocyte. It is not uncommon to observe two follicles developing to approximately 10 mm, with one becoming dominant and growing and the other regressing. LH reinitiates meiosis of the oocyte and typically ovulation occurs within 36 hours of its "surge" in circulating levels. Estradiol is synthesized by the granulosa cells and provides important feedback to the pituitary in the production of FSH and LH.

Beginning with menarche, during spontaneous cycles there usually is development of one or sometimes two dominant follicles. TVS can depict the developing follicles starting when they measure between 3 and 5 mm. In the spontaneous cycle, usually there is one or at the most two follicles that develop to measure approximately 10 mm in size. As the follicle matures, more fluid is elaborated into its center, and the number of granulosa cells lining the inner wall of the follicle increases. The oocyte, which is less than a tenth of a millimeter, is surrounded by a cluster of granulosa cells. This complex is termed the cumulus oophorus. It measures approximately 1 mm and occasionally can be depicted along the wall of some mature follicles with TVS. Immediately before ovulation the cumulus separates from the wall and floats freely within the center of the follicle. Even with the enhanced resolution afforded by TVS, the attached or floating cumulus is only rarely visualized.

Mature follicles (ones that contain a mature oocyte) typically measure from 17 to 25 mm in average inner dimension (Fleischer et al, 1981) (Fig. 6-1). Within the same individual, however, the size of a mature follicle is relatively constant cycle to cycle. Intrafollicular echoes may be observed with mature follicles, probably arising from clusters of granulosa cells that shear off the wall near the time of ovulation. After ovulation, the follicular wall becomes irregular as the follicle becomes "deflated" (Figs. 6-2, 6-3). The fresh corpus luteum usually appears as a hypoechoic structure with an irregular wall and may contain some internal echoes corresponding to hemorrhage. As the corpus luteum develops 4 to 8 days after ovulation, it appears as an echogenic structure of approximately 15 mm. Its wall is thickened by the process of luteinization (see Fig. 6-3).

In addition to delineation of changes in follicle size and morphology, TVS can depict the presence of intraperitoneal fluid (Fig. 6-4). It is normal to have approximately 1 to 3 ml in the cul-de-sac throughout the cycle. When ovulation occurs, there is typically between 4 and 5 ml of fluid within the cul-de-sac. The intraperitoneal fluid resulting from ovulation may be loculated outside of the posterior cul-de-sac, surrounding bowel loops in the lower abdomen and upper pelvis, or in the anterior cul-de-sac superior to the uterine fundus.

INDUCED OVULATION

In patients whose infertility can be attributed to an ovulation abnormality, ovulation induction is indicated. Ovulation induction is also used in in vitro fertilization-embryo transfer (IVF-ET) to increase the number of oocytes aspirated, which in turn increases the number of fertilized concepti that may be transferred, thereby increasing the chance of pregnancy.

The two medications most commonly used for ovulation induction include clomiphene citrate (CC) and human menopausal gonadotropin (hMG). Although both medications result in the development of multiple follicles, they act by different mechanisms. TVS has a vital role in monitoring follicular development in women receiving ovulation-induction medication (Ritchie, 1986; Tarlatizis et al, 1984).

Patients undergoing ovulation induction are usually examined every other day beginning between days 7 and 9. For patients undergoing IVF-ET, patients begin to be examined by TVS earlier in their cycles and usually daily in an attempt to carefully monitor their follicular development.

CC is considered an estrogen antagonist and exerts its effect by binding estrogen receptor sites in the pituitary and hypothalamus. This leads to increased FSH secretion by the pituitary, thereby recruiting more follicles. Since the process of selection and dominance may be overridden, multiple, relatively synchronous follicles usually develop (Fig. 6-5). Although the preovulatory E_2-LH feedback may be intact in CC-treated patients with an intact hypothalamus, some patients are given human chorionic gonadotropin (hCG) to induce final follicular and oocyte maturation.

Follicular development with CC can be different than that observed in spontaneous cycles. Specifically, each follicle seems to develop at an individual rate and at times may be accelerated or slowed down. Therefore the largest follicle on a given date may not be the same 2 days later and may not even be the one that is most mature. Furthermore, correlation of E_2 and follicle sizes is poor, and the maximum preovulatory diameter can range from 19 to 24 mm.

Unlike CC, treatment with hMG does not require an intact hypothalamus or pituitary. In hMG-treated patients, there seem to be two distinct patterns of follicular development (Ritchie, 1986). In those amenorrheic women with no exogenous estrogen, estrogenic activity, and dormant ovaries, the response to endogenous gonadotropins is to develop a small number of large follicles (see Fig. 6-4). The growth rate and E_2

secretion are linear, correlate well, and are of equal predictive value. A high pregnancy rate is achieved in this group. In contrast, patients with estrogenic activity who harbor antral follicles at different stages of development react differently (Fig. 6-6). Stimulation of these patients requires less hMG and usually results in the rapid recruitment of many follicles with different growth rates in varying degrees of E_2 secretory capacity. Also, the rate at which E_2 increases is exponential, increasing the risk of hyperstimulation. Thus, there is a dissociation between follicle size and E_2 levels, suggesting that growth rate and functional maturity are asynchronous. This group of women particularly benefits from combined E_2 and follicular monitoring with TVS. Because hMG contains both FSH and LH and a spontaneous LH surge is less frequent when inducing follicular development with hMG, hCG may be required to induce final follicular maturation. TVS delineation of follicle size is crucial since hCG is best administered once follicles reach 15 to 18 mm in size.

For in vitro fertilization, follicles are typically aspirated when they reach 15 to 18 mm in average dimension and when there is evidence by estradiol values of a mature follicle (approximately 400 pg/mL/mature follicle) (Marrs et al, 1983). Another sonographic sign of a mature follicle is the presence of low-level, intrafollicular echoes. These echoes probably arise from clumps of granulosa cells that have separated from the follicular wall. In one study involving patients who underwent ovulation induction and were scanned transabdominally, a higher pregnancy rate was achieved in those patients whose follicles demonstrated these intrafollicular echoes (Mendelson et al, 1985).

TVS has an important role in decreasing the likelihood of ovarian hyperstimulation. Ovarian hyperstimulation disorder occurs in various degrees of severity in most patients who undergo ovulation induction, ranging from mild abdominal discomfort (probably due to the distension of the ovarian capsule) to severe circulatory compromise and electrolyte imbalance (probably secondary to ascites and/or pleural effusions that may develop). The more severe form, ovarian hyperstimulation syndrome (OHSS), is usually associated with massive stromal edema of the ovary. The enlarged ovaries may be prone to torsion. The symptoms associated with OHSS usually begin 5 to 8 days after hCG is given but can be most severe in patients who actually achieve pregnancy. Recent studies have shown that hyperstimulation is unlikely in women whose ovaries contain several large (over 15 mm) follicles and tends to occur when there are several small or intermediately sized follicles (Blankstein et al, 1987).

Although sonographic findings of bilaterally enlarged ovaries that have multiple immature follicles with the presence of intraperitoneal fluid may suggest the possibility of hyperstimulation, this syndrome can be more accurately predicted by extremely high levels of E_2 (over 3000 pg/mL). Despite the superovulation required for IVF, hyperstimulation is only rarely encountered. This is probably a reflection of the close monitoring that these patients receive but also may be secondary to drainage and collapse of the aspirated follicles.

On TVS, patients with OHSS usually have bilaterally enlarged ovaries (over 10 cm) that may contain several hypoechoic areas (Fig. 6-7). The hypoechoic areas may correspond to atretic follicles or regions of hemorrhage within the ovary. Because it demonstrates lack of arterial and venous flow, color Doppler sonography may be useful in the detection of ovarian torsion (see Fig. 6-7). One should realize that the ovary has a dual blood supply, however: one arising from the adnexal branch of the uterine artery; the other coursing through the infundibulopelvic ligament (Fig. 6-8). Torsion may affect one arterial blood supply more than the other, resulting in the presence of arterial flow on color Doppler.

The pregnancies that occur with OHSS may be early (<4 weeks), and no definitive sonographic findings may be found. Intraperitoneal fluid is usually present and is a consequence of the serum osmotic imbalance. With supportive medical therapy, this syndrome usually spontaneously regresses.

After induced ovulation, the stimulated follicles usually undergo regression but may persist and enlarge over the remainder of the cycle. This seems to be most commonly seen in patients on gonadotropin releasing hormone (GnRH) analogs. The presence of physiologic ovarian cysts (over 3 cm) may preclude attempts at ovulation induction during that cycle since the previously induced follicles may not have totally regressed and the remaining ovarian tissue may not be as responsive to ovulation-induction medication. Theoretically the risk of torsion and rupture may also be increased in these women.

TVS can also detect other adnexal masses such as a hydrosalpinx, endometriomas, paraovarian cysts, or peritoneal cysts that may mimic physiologic cysts or follicles that are either totally anechoic or contain low-level homogeneous echoes. These masses can be differentiated from ovarian cysts since they are extraovarian.

Sonographic monitoring of follicular development is also helpful in decreasing the likelihood of multiple gestations that may occur with fertilization of multiple ova. It is difficult to predict which pregnancies will result in multiple births, however. Clearly, however, when there are more than four mature follicles, the chance for multiple gestation beyond twinning is more probable than if only two or three mature follicles are induced.

Guided Procedures

There has been development of needle guides which can be attached to transvaginal probes and greatly facilitate guided follicular aspiration. After the probe is draped with a condom, these needle guides can be placed directly on the transducer-probe, allowing for a direct and continuous visualization of the aspirating needle as it is advanced into the ovary (Fig. 6-9). The "line of sight" is generated on the monitor and closely approximates the needle path that will be traversed.

FOLLICULAR ASPIRATION

TVS-guided follicular aspiration is the preferred procedure of choice for oocyte retrieval over the previously used laparoscopic techniques. The major advantages to this technique include decreased exposure to general anesthesia, lower chance for operative complications, and feasibility of performing this procedure in an outpatient setting. The success rate, as determined by the number of fertilizable oocytes retrieved and pregnancies produced, is comparable with the laparoscopic technique (Feldberg et al, 1988) (Table 6-1). The procedure is also advantageous in patients with pelvic adhesions since laparoscopic access to the ovary may be hampered (Taylor et al, 1986). Most importantly, acceptance of the procedure by patients is high (Schulman et al, 1987; Feichtinger and Kemeter, 1986; Hammarberg et al, 1987).

There are several methods for follicular aspiration

that involve sonographic guidance (Schulman et al, 1987; Feichtinger and Kemeter, 1986; Hammarberg et al, 1987; Dellenbach et al, 1985; Parsons et al, 1985; Marrs, 1986) (Fig. 6-10). These include TVS for guidance of transvaginal aspiration, transabdominal sonography for guidance of transvaginal aspiration, transabdominal sonography for guidance of transvesical aspiration, and transabdominal sonographic guidance for transurethral aspiration. Although TVS with transvaginal aspiration is used most frequently, the actual method used may be tailored to each patient according to the anatomic position of the ovary and other structures. For example, the transvaginal aspiration is the preferred route when the ovaries are in the cul-de-sac, whereas the per urethral approach may be used for aspiration of follicles in ovaries located near the dome of the bladder.

With all of these aspiration techniques, a long (30 cm) 16- or 18-gauge needle that is scored at the tip is used, which results in its enhanced sonographic visualization (see Fig. 6-9D). The aspiration procedure is performed under local anesthesia and with supplemental intravenous or intramuscular medication.

For transvaginal aspiration with transvaginal transducers, a needle guide is attached to the transducer-probe (see Fig. 6-9). This allows the needle to traverse in the beam path of the transducer (see Fig. 6-9). The cursor is displayed on the scanner's screen, which indicates the path of the needle. After a condom containing sterile gel is placed over the transducer and the sterile needle guide attached, the operator manipulates the transducer to optimally delineate the ovary (see Fig. 6-10A). The desired follicle is brought into the line of sight and the needle is introduced into the needle guide. After the initial aspiration, the follicle is filled with buffered media and flushed so that chances for retrieving a mature oocyte are maximized (see Fig. 6-10B,C).

This aspiration technique has been associated with

Table 6-1   Results of Ovum Pickup by Three Methods

	Laparoscopic	Transvesical	Transvaginal
Oocytes recovered/patient	6.4 ± 0.9	6.2 ± 0.3	5.7 ± 0.6
Oocytes recovered/follicle (%)	93.0	86.0	82.0
Fertilization rate (%)	73.6	72.3	70.9
Cleavage rate (%)	82.6	79.4	81.6
Number of embryos transferred	3.9 ± 0.6	3.2 ± 6.4	3.6 ± 0.3
Pregnancy rate/per pickup (%)	23.7	22.3	21.6
Pregnancy rate/transfer (%)	26.6	26.7	25.9
Pregnancy rate/cycle (%)	20.2	22.6	21.1

From Feldberg D, Goldman JA, Ashkenazi J, et al. Transvaginal oocyte retrieval controlled by vaginal probe for in vitro fertilization: a comparative study. *J Ultrasound Med* 1988; 7:339–343.

a low complication rate. One complication that has been described is inadvertent introduction of the needle into a vessel (usually the internal iliac vein) in the pelvis (Feldberg et al, 1988). This problem can be avoided if the operator carefully exams any round structure in both long- and short-axis to identify a vascular structure from a follicle.

The use of GnRH analogs (Lupron) may be associated with the development of follicular cysts. It is thought that the presence of the cysts may impair folliculogenesis because of either the elaboration of hormones or a direct affect on reducing perfusion by parenchymal compression by the cyst itself. In these cases, TVS-guided aspiration affords direct visualization and monitoring of guidance for aspiration of these physiologic cysts (Fig. 6-11A,B).

GUIDED TUBAL CANNULATION

TVS is being used for transcervical cannulization of the uterine and tubal lumen (Jansen and Anderson, 1987). A technique for sonographic guidance of placement of a catheter into the fallopian tubes for gamete intrafallopian transfer (GIFT) procedure has been described (Fig. 6-12) and has several advantages over hysteroscopically guided tubal cannulation (Jansen and Anderson, 1987). For this procedure, a catheter is placed transcervically and manipulated into the area of the uterine cornu. The catheter is slowly introduced under sonographic guidance into the tubal ostia. Once the catheter is in the distal isthmic portion of the fallopian tube, the sperm and ova may be introduced through the cannula directly into the tube.

Endometrial Assessment

Besides the factors involved in obtaining a fertilized ovum, the developmental state of the endometrium may also be a factor influencing the probability that conception will occur (Rabinowitz et al, 1986). Since the endometrium can also be delineated during examinations performed for follicular monitoring, several investigators have evaluated this specialized mucus membrane in an attempt to study whether there is an optimal thickness or texture (Fleischer et al, 1986; Thickman et al, 1986; Glissant et al, 1985; Fleischer et al, 1984). There is a clear association of the sonographic texture of the endometrium and the circulating levels of estrogen and progesterone (Rabinowitz et al, 1986).

In spontaneous and induced cycles, the sonographic appearance of the endometrium varies according to its specific phases of development. In the menstrual phase, the endometrium appears as a thin, broken echogenic interface. In the proliferative phase, it thickens and becomes isoechoic, measuring 3 to 5 mm in anteroposterior width. Its relative hypoechogenicity is related to the relatively orderly organization of the glandular elements within the endometrium. As ovulation approaches, the endometrium becomes more echogenic; this is probably related to development of secretions within the endometrial glands and the numerous interfaces that arise from distended and tortuous glands. In the peri-ovulatory period, there usually is a hypoechoic area within the inner endometrium that most likely represents edema of the compactum layer. This finding has been described as a means of confirming that ovulation has occurred, however, with TVS this finding has been observed both before and immediately after ovulation. During the secretory phase, the endometrium achieves its greatest thickness (between 6 and 12 mm) and echogenicity. In addition to the echogenic endometrium, a hypoechoic band beneath the endometrium can be identified, probably arising from the inner layer of the myometrium.

The fact that medications used for ovulation induction may alter the development of the endometrium has been shown by both sonographic and histologic studies (Fleischer et al, 1984). The relative importance of these changes relative to success or failure of achieving pregnancy is only speculative, however. One study evaluated the endometrial thickness (includes both layers) in the secretory phase showed that conception was unlikely in endometria that measured less than 13 mm 11 days after ovulation (Fleischer et al, 1984). Other studies have indicated that the texture of the endometrium may be related to the success or failure of pregnancy, but no statistical predictive value could be obtained from these various patterns (Rabinowitz et al, 1986; Glissant et al, 1985). Other studies involved in sonographic evaluation of endometrium during ovulation induction have failed to demonstrate any specific changes in its thickness associated with success or failure to achieve pregnancy (Rabinowitz et al, 1986; Glissant et al, 1985). Our studies using TVS have indicated that there is a statistically significant difference in the pregnancy rate when the endometrium has a multi-layered appearance (Fig. 6-13). In two groups of 20 patients that underwent similar but not identical stimulations, 27% of the nonconception group showed a multilayered endometrium versus 79% of the group that conceived. This was statistically different even though the number of mature follicles, E_2 values, and number of transferred embryos were not (Table 6-2, Fig. 6-13).

TVS may have a role in further evaluation of patients who have luteal phase inadequacy. It is conceivable that these patients have underdeveloped endometria that could be characterized sonographically as thinner and less echoic than expected.

Table 6-2 Conception Versus Nonconception IVF Groups

	Endometrial Width (mm) (mean ± SD)	Change Over 4 d (mm)	Percent Multi-layered	Mature Number of Follicles >1.5 cm	E₂ (pg/mL)	Number of Retrieved Ova	Number of Embryo Transferred
Nonconception	9.5 ± 1.0	3.1	27	3.1	1,157	3.3	2.3
Conception	9.8 ± 0.9	1.6	74	3.1	1,137	4.1	2.1
P value	NS	.05	.0001	NS	NS	.05	NS

NS, not significant.

Other Applications

TVS has a role secondary to hysterosalpingography in the evaluation of certain uterine malformations and tubal disorders. Malformed uteri can be characterized sonographically by delineation of the echogenic secretory phase endometrium within the uterine lumen. Hematometra may result from cervical and/or lower uterine malformations. Bicornuate uterus may be difficult to distinguish from septated uterus in the nongravid state. Uterine septa are readily apparent as a thick intraluminal interface in a gravid uterus, however, sometimes separating the fetus and placenta.

The precise location of an intrauterine contraceptive device (IUD) relative to the uterine lumen can also be determined sonographically, particularly with the use of TVS (Fig. 6-14A,B). The location of the IUD relative to a gestational sac may figure in the decision of whether or not to attempt removal of the IUD. If an IUD is inferior to the sac, attempts at removal may be feasible.

TVS can be used to delineate enlarged and dilated fallopian tubes and establish their relationship to the ovary (Fig. 6-14C). The nondistended fallopian tube can be recognized only occasionally. On TVS, the area of the proximal tube can be identified by the endometrium that projects into the area of the uterine cornu. An injectable contrast medium has been developed that clearly demonstrates tubal patency, especially when monitored with color Doppler sonography.

Sonography also has an important role in evaluating women with infertility who eventually become pregnant. These women have a higher incidence of ectopic pregnancy, anembryonic pregnancy, and spontaneous abortion. Clinical suspicion of these conditions is clearly an indication for TVS evaluation.

Future Applications

The transducer used for TVS can be capable of simultaneous imaging and pulsed Doppler assessment of uterine and adnexal vasculature. Specifically, the ascending branch of the uterine artery can be assessed with pulsed Doppler. The information obtained can reveal uterine and adnexal perfusion and is extremely important in excluding the possibility of adnexal torsion. As in other parenchymal organs, the waveform and resistance can be related to physiologic activity. For example, corpus luteum function is characterized by diastolic flow as opposed to sharp systolic peaks and no diastolic flow characteristic of ovaries is seen in the quiescent state. The adequacy of corpus luteum development may be assessed using this method. Similarly, pulsed Doppler capabilities within the vaginal probe may allow assessment of uterine perfusion, which may be related to relative chance of conception.

Fingertip probes may allow more enhanced visualization of the uterus and ovary than that afforded by conventional TVS imaging.

Summary

TVS affords accurate follicular monitoring and guidance for follicular aspiration. It can also assess endometrial development and provide a means for physiologic assessment of adnexal and uterine blood flow.

References

Blankstein J, Shalev J, Saadon T, et al. Ovarian hyperstimulation syndrome: prediction by number and size of preovulatory ovarian follicles. *Fertil Steril* 1987;47:597–602.

Dellenbach P, Nisand I, Moreau L, et al. Transvaginal sonographically controlled follicle puncture for oocyte retrieval. *Fertil Steril* 1985;44:656.

Feichtinger W, Kemeter P. Ultrasound-guided aspiration of human ovarian follicles for *in vitro* fertilization. In: Sanders RC, Hill M, eds: *Ultrasound Annual*. New York: Raven Press, 1986:25–39.

Feldberg D, Goldman JA, Ashkenazi J, et al. Transvaginal oocyte retrieval controlled by vaginal probe for in vitro fertilization: a comparative study. *J Ultrasound Med* 1988;7:339–343.

Fleischer AC, Daniell JF, Rodier J, et al. Sonographic monitoring of ovarian follicular development. *J Clin Ultrasound* 1981;9:275–280.

Fleischer AC, Pittaway DE, Wentz AC, et al. The uses of sonography for monitoring ovarian follicular development. In: Sanders RC, Hill M, eds. *Ultrasound Annual*. New York: Raven Press, 1983:163–205.

Fleischer AC, Pittaway DE, Beard LA, et al. Sonographic depiction of endometrial changes occurring with ovulation induction. *J Ultrasound Med* 1984;3:341–346.

Fleischer AC, Herbert CM, Sacks GA, et al. Sonography of the endometrium during conception and nonconception cycles of *in vitro* fertilization and embryo transfer. *Fertil Steril* 1986;46:442.

Geisthovel F, Skubsch U, Zabel G, et al. Ultrasonographic and hormonal studies in physiologic and insufficient menstrual cycles. *Fertil Steril* 1983;39:277.

Glissant A, de Mouzon J, Frydman R. Ultrasound study of the endometrium during *in vitro* fertilization cycles. *Fertil Steril* 1985;44:786.

Hammarberg K, Enk L, Nilsson L, et al. Oocyte retrieval under the guidance of a vaginal transducer: evaluation of patient acceptance. *Hum Reprod* 1987;2:487–490.

Hann LE, Hall DA, McArdle CR, et al. Polycystic ovarian disease: sonographic spectrum. *Radiology* 1984;150:531.

Hilgers TW, Dvorak AD, Tamisiea DF, et al. Sonographic definition of the empty follicle syndrome. *J Ultrasound Med* 1989;8:411–416.

Jansen RPS, Anderson JC. Catheterisation of the fallopian tubes from the vagina. *Lancet* 1987;2:309–310.

Liukkonen S, Koskimies AI, Tenhunen A, et al. Diagnosis of luteinized unruptured follicle (LUF) syndrome by ultrasound. *Fertil Steril* 1984;41:26. Abstract.

Marrs RP, Vargyas JM, March CM. Correlation of ultrasonic and endocrinologic measurements in human menopausal gonadotropin therapy. *Am J Obstet Gynecol* 1983;145:417.

Marrs RP. Does the method of oocyte collection have a major influence on *in vitro* fertilization? *Fertil Steril* 1986;46:193–195.

McArdle CR, Seibel M, Weinstein F, et al. Induction of ovulation monitored by ultrasound. *Radiology* 1983;148:809–812.

Mendelson EB, Friedman H, Neiman HL, et al. The role of imaging in infertility management. *AJR* 1985;144:415–420.

Parsons J, Booker M, Goswamy R, et al. Oocyte retrieval for in-vitro fertilisation by ultrasonically guided needle aspiration via the urethra. *Lancet* 1985;1:1076–1077.

Rabinowitz R, Laufer N, Lewin A, et al. The value of ultrasonographic endometrial measurement in the prediction of pregnancy following *in vitro* fertilization. *Fertil Steril* 1986;45:824.

Ritchie WGM. Sonographic evaluation of normal and induced ovulation. *Radiology* 1986;161:1–10.

Schulman JD, Dorfmann AD, Jones SL, et al. Outpatient *in vitro* fertilization using transvaginal ultrasound-guided oocyte retrieval. *Obstet Gynecol* 1987;69:665–668.

Tarlatizis BC, Laufer N, DeCherney AH. The use of ovarian ultrasonography in monitoring ovulation induction. *J In Vitro Fert Embryo Transfer* 1984;1:226–232.

Taylor PJ, Wiseman D, Mahadevan M, et al. "Ultrasound rescue": a successful alternative form of oocyte recovery in patients with periovarian adhesions. *Am J Obstet Gynecol* 1986;154:240–244.

Thickman D, Arger P, Tureck R, et al. Sonographic assessment of the endometrium in patients undergoing *in vitro* fertilization. *J Ultrasound Med* 1986;5:197–201.

Winfield AC, Fleischer AC, Moore DE. Diagnostic imaging in infertility. *Curr Probl Diagn Radiol* 1990;19:1–38.

FIGURE 6-1   TVS Showing a Mature Follicle Within Left Ovary

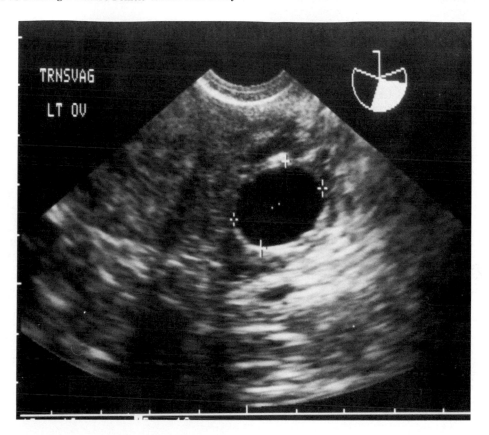

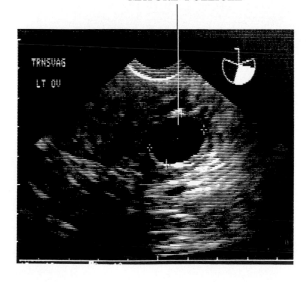

MATURE FOLLICLE

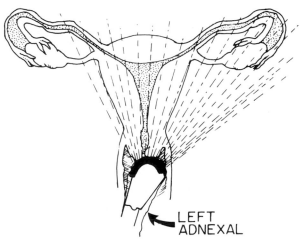

LEFT
ADNEXAL

FIGURE 6-2   Postovulatory Follicle During a Spontaneous Cycle with Thickened, Serrated Wall

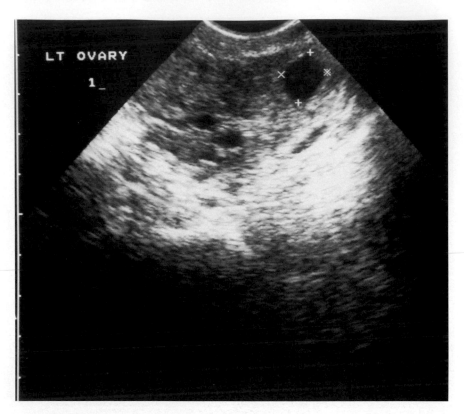

CORPUS LUTEUM

LEFT ADNEXAL

FIGURE 6-3 TVS Mimics of a Follicle

6-3A Rounded cystic structure near the left ovary representing a paraovarian cyst.

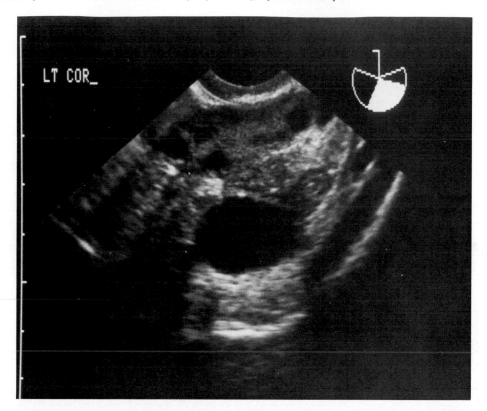

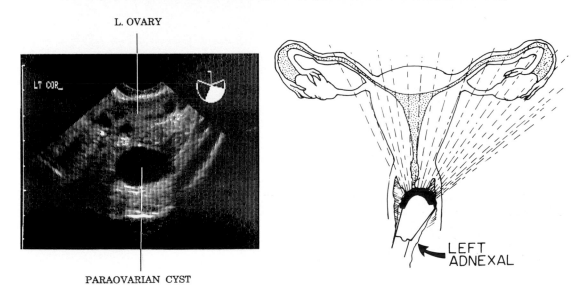

(continued)

FIGURE 6-3   TVS Mimics of a Follicle *(continued)*

6-3B   Fluid-filled small bowel adjacent to the right ovary.

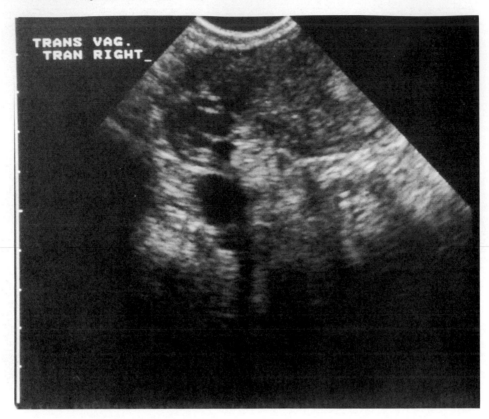

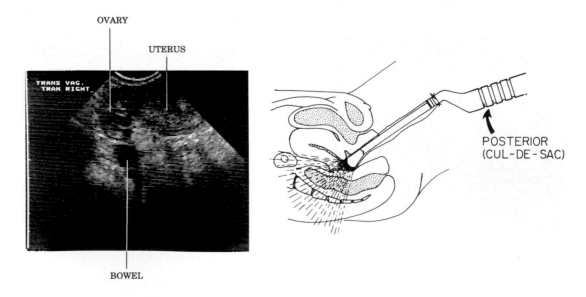

FIGURE 6-4   Intraperitoneal Fluid After Ovulation

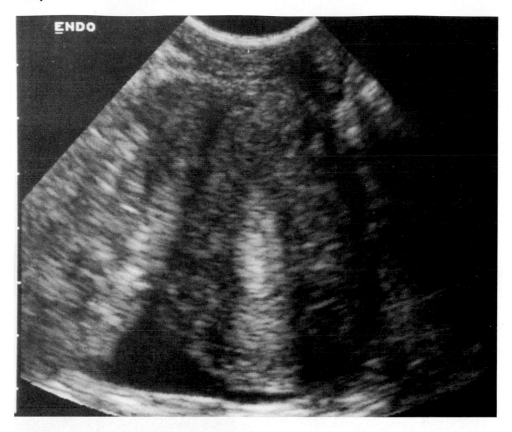

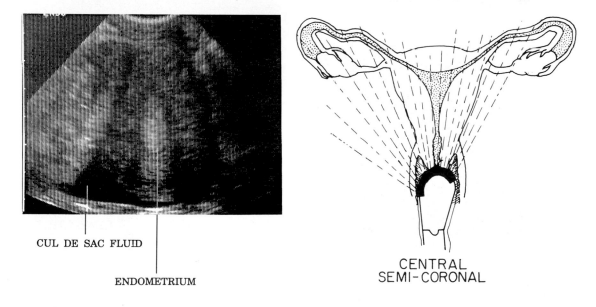

CUL DE SAC FLUID

ENDOMETRIUM

CENTRAL
SEMI-CORONAL

FIGURE 6-5   Multiple Mature Follicles Resulting from Clomid Ovulation Induction. A cumulus is seen in the measured follicle.

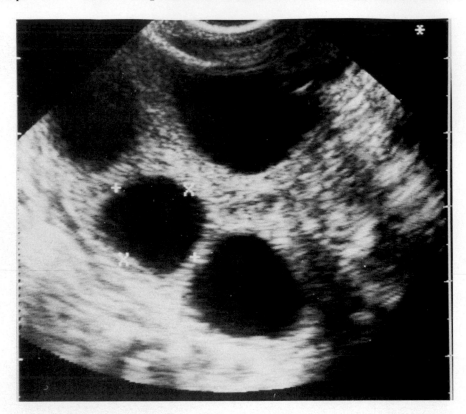

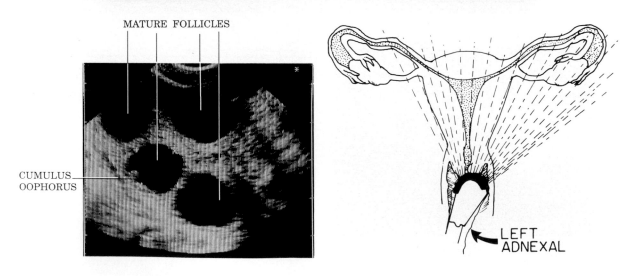

MATURE FOLLICLES

CUMULUS OOPHORUS

LEFT ADNEXAL

FIGURE 6-6   Multiple Follicles at Various Stages of Development

6-6A   Polycystic ovary with development of single dominant follicle.

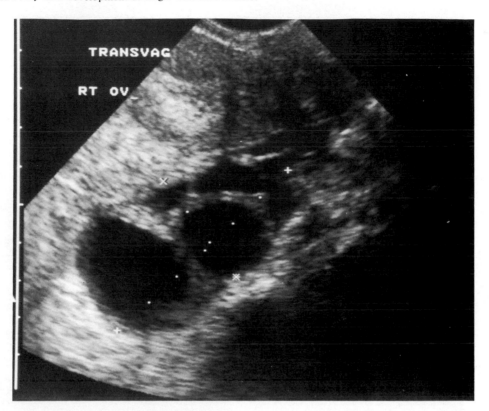

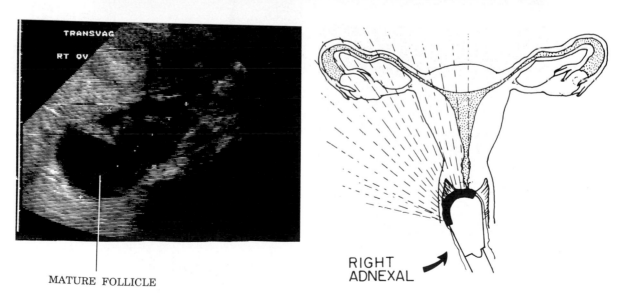

MATURE FOLLICLE

RIGHT
ADNEXAL

(continued)

FIGURE 6-6   Multiple Follicles at Various Stages of Development *(continued)*

6-6B   Ovary containing several immature follicles. In one, the granulosa cell layer is separating.

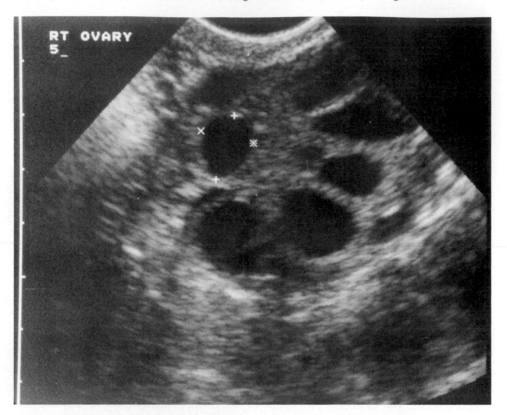

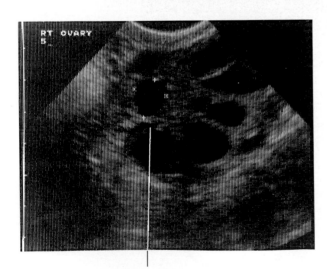

SEPARATING GRANULOSA CELL LAYER

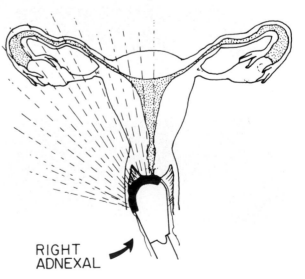

RIGHT
ADNEXAL

FIGURE 6-7   OHSS

6-7A   Enlarged right ovary with numerous follicles. Duplex Doppler shows arterial flow within the ovary, thus excluding torsion.

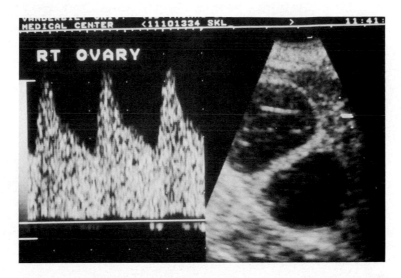

6-7B   Enlarged left ovary with numerous follicles. Arterial flow is shown as in the right ovary.

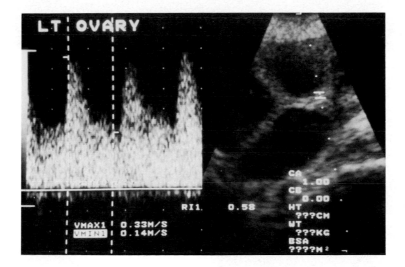

FIGURE 6-8 Paracervical Vessels

6-8A Distended paracervical vessels that should be avoided during aspiration procedures.

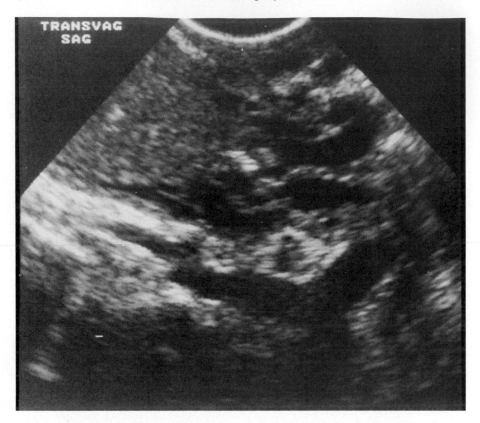

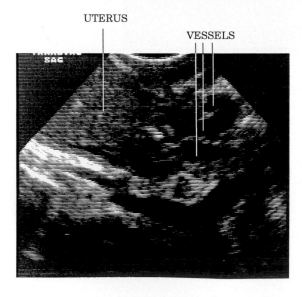

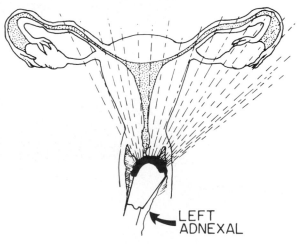

FIGURE 6-8   Paracervical Vessels *(continued)*

6-8B   Uterine arteries adjacent to the cervix.

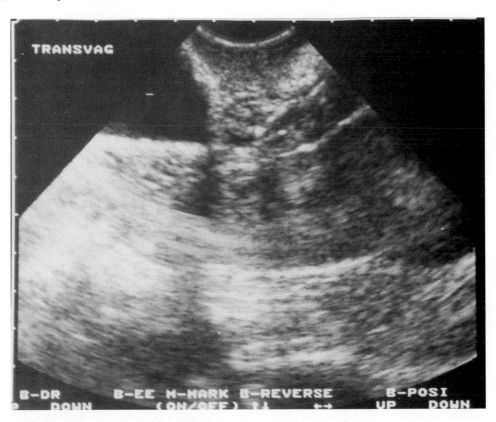

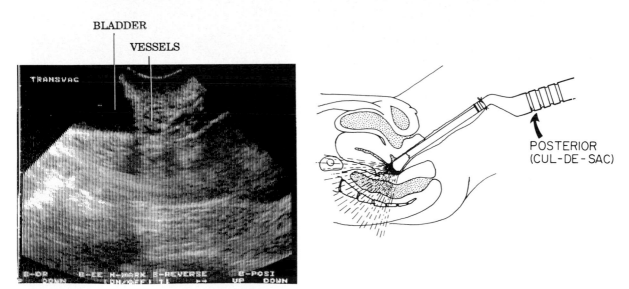

FIGURE 6-9   Guided Procedures. *A*. Draped probe with needle guide attached. *B*. Diagram of guided transvaginal follicle aspiration. *C*. Display on monitor showing path of needle. *D*. Needle showing scored tip.

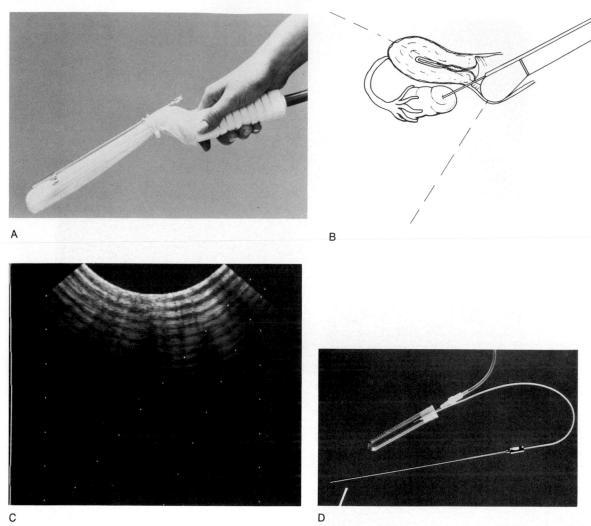

A

B

C

D

FIGURE 6-10   Guided Follicular Aspiration

6-10A   Before aspiration. The desired follicle is aligned within the beam path.

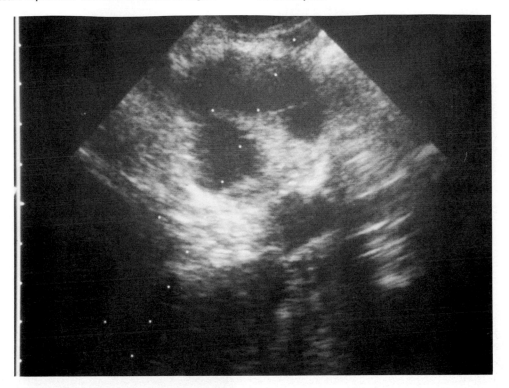

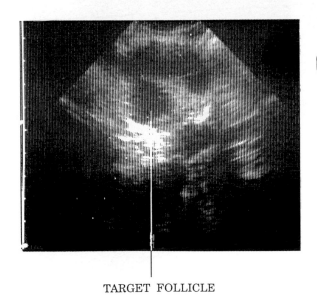

TARGET FOLLICLE

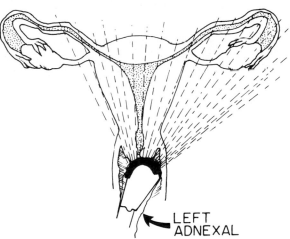

LEFT
ADNEXAL

(continued)

FIGURE 6-10   Guided Follicular Aspiration (*continued*)

6-10B   After aspiration the echogenic needle tip can be seen within the aspirated follicle.

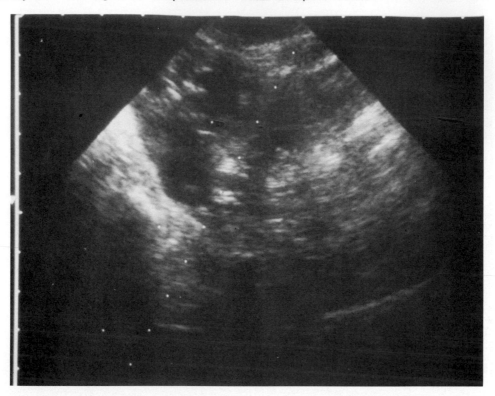

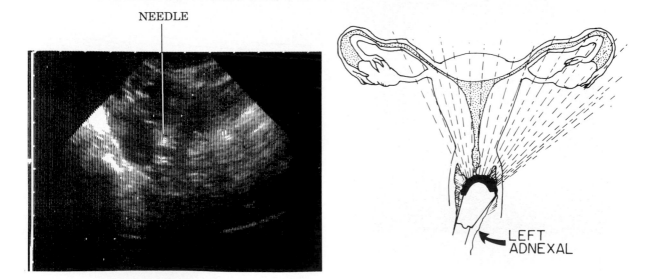

FIGURE 6-10   Guided Follicular Aspiration *(continued)*

6-10C   Needle guided into follicle adjacent to a hydrosalpinx.

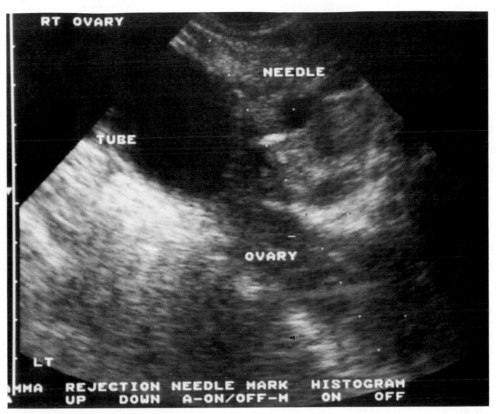

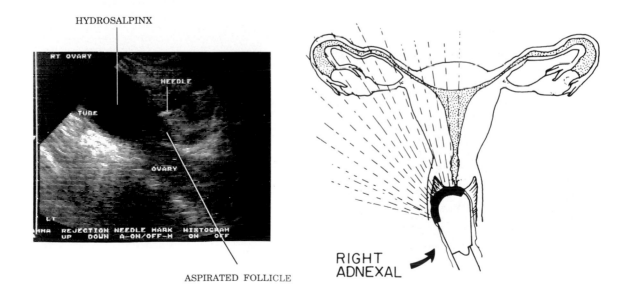

FIGURE 6-11   Cyst Aspiration Associated with Lupron Cycle

6-11A   Needle tip within cyst.

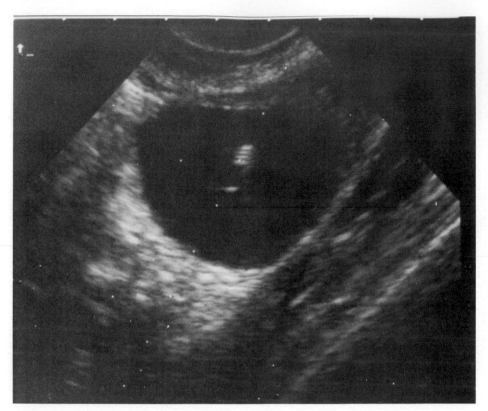

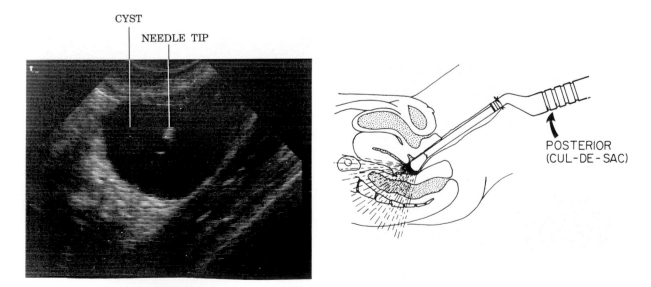

FIGURE 6-11   Cyst Aspiration Associated with Lupron Cycle *(continued)*

6-11B   After aspiration.

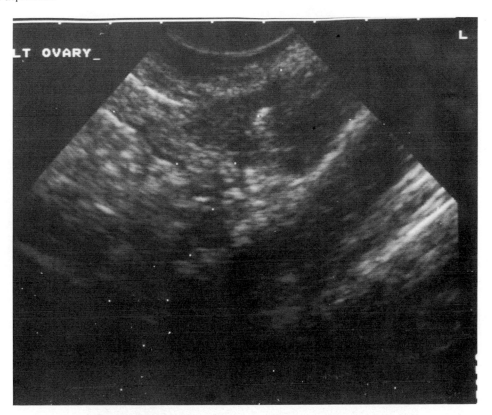

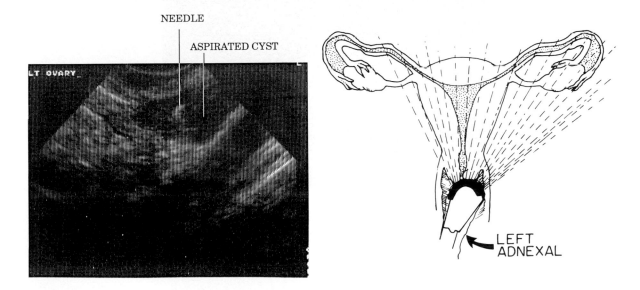

FIGURE 6-12   Tubal Cannulation

6-12A   Diagram of TVS guidance.

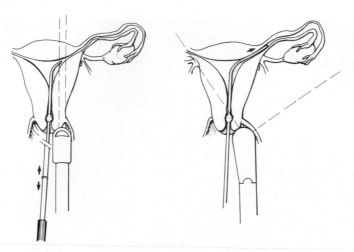

6-12B   Cannula through ostia.

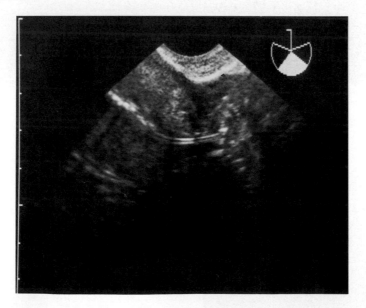

FIGURE 6-12   **Tubal Cannulation** *(continued)*

6-12C   Inner catheter advanced into isthmic portion of tube.

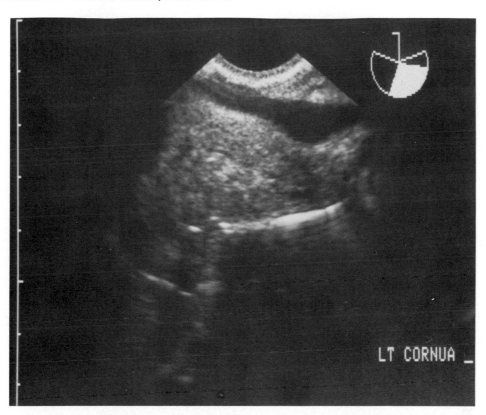

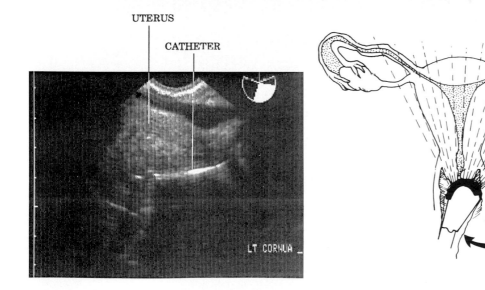

(continued)

FIGURE 6-12   Tubal Cannulation *(continued)*

6-12D   Radiograph of opened tube after dilation.

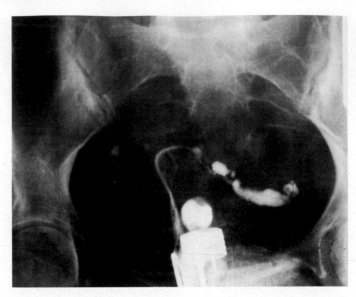

FIGURE 6-13   **Endometrial Development. The uterus is shown in sagittal plane, long-axis view.**

6-13A   Proliferative phase; endometrium isoechoic to myometrium.

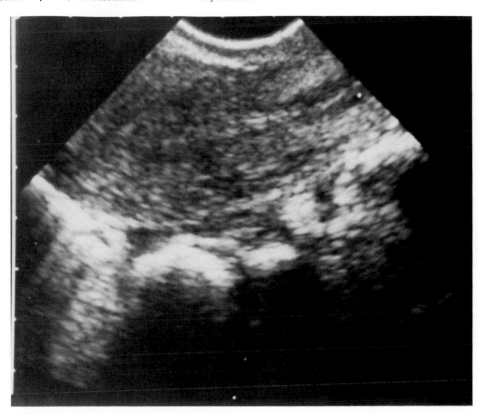

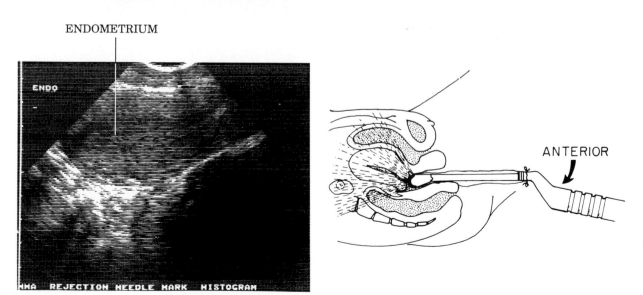

(continued)

FIGURE 6-13   **Endometrial Development. The uterus is shown in sagittal plane, long-axis view** *(continued).*

6-13B   Late proliferative, periovulatory phase showing multilayers.

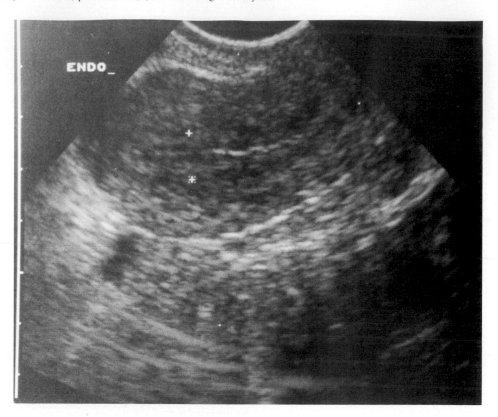

ENDOMETRIUM

CENTRAL
SAGITTAL

FIGURE 6-13   Endometrial Development. The uterus is shown in sagittal plane, long-axis view *(continued)*.

6-13C   Secretory phase, uniformly echogenic and thick endometrium.

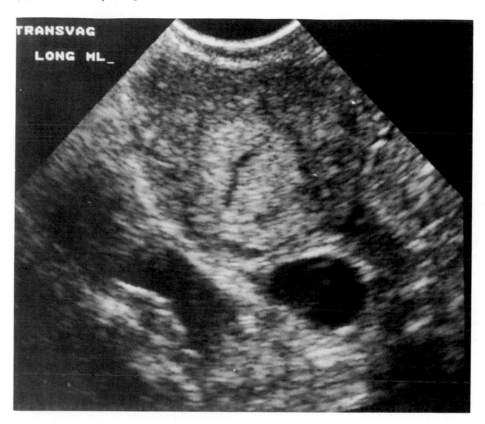

SECRETORY ENDOMETRIUM

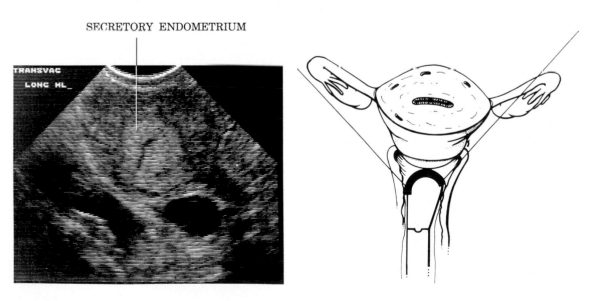

FIGURE 6-14   Miscellaneous Applications

6-14A   CU-7 IUD within upper uterine lumen.

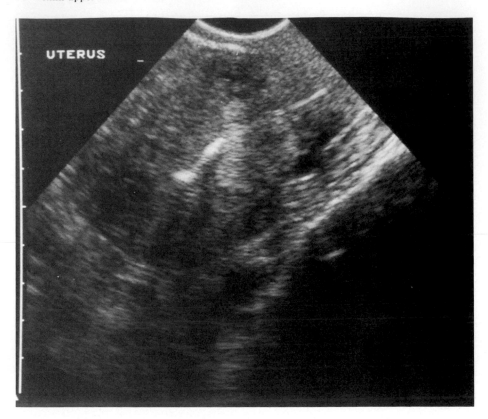

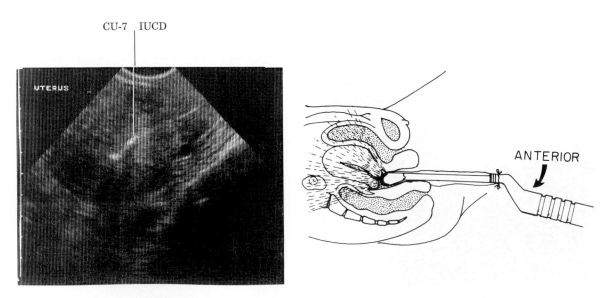

FIGURE 6-14   **Miscellaneous Applications** *(continued)*

6-14B   CU-7 IUD in lower corpus, upper cervix.

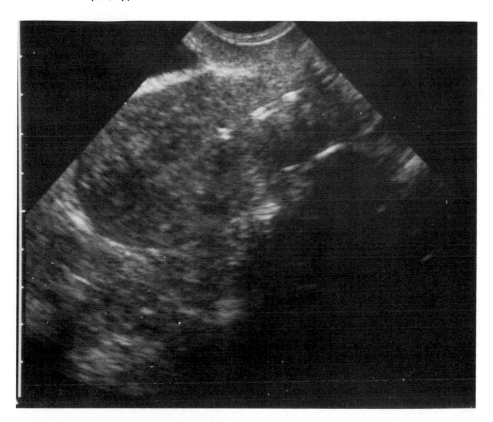

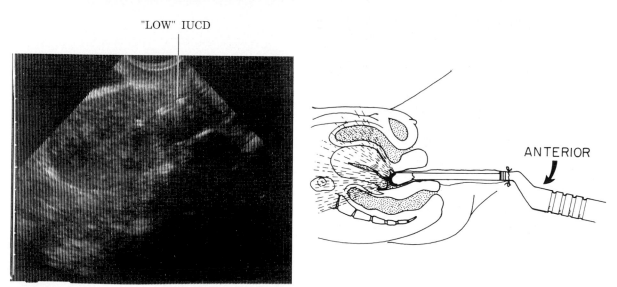

(continued)

FIGURE 6-14   **Miscellaneous Applications** *(continued)*

6-14C   Hydrosalpinx (between cursors) of right tube.

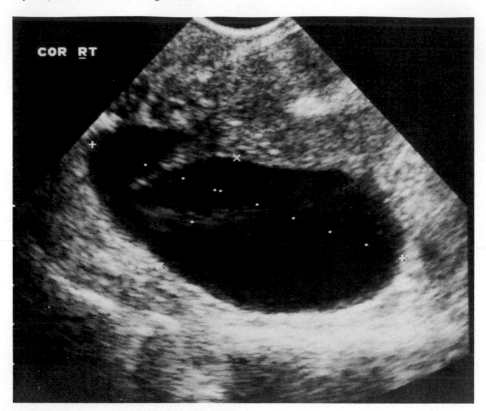

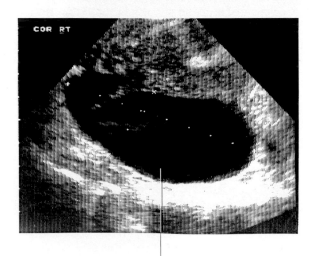

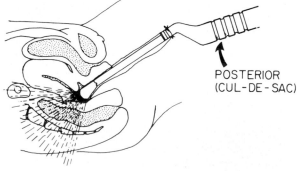

HYDROSALPINX

POSTERIOR
(CUL-DE-SAC)

Chapter 7

Normal Early Pregnancy

Arthur C. Fleischer, MD
Bhaskara K. Rao, MD
Donna M. Kepple, RDMS

Introduction

Transvaginal sonography (TVS) affords detailed delineation of the anatomic changes that occur in the first trimester of pregnancy. In general, definitive sonographic findings such as the presence or absence of a gestational sac and the presence or absence of an embryo/fetus with or without heart motion can be established 1 week before confirmation by conventional transabdominal scanning techniques (Pennell et al, 1987). Certain anatomic "milestones" can predictably be seen with TVS (Table 7-1).

TVS Milestones

One of the earliest sonographic findings in intrauterine pregnancy is the thickening of the decidua that occurs at approximately 3 to 4 weeks (Fig. 7-1). After 4 weeks, a small (3 to 5 mm) hypoechoic area surrounded by an echogenic rim can be seen within the choriodecidual tissue. This is the chorionic sac (Fig. 7-2). The sac usually enlarges from 3 to 10 mm in average dimension and grows at a rate of 1 to 1.1 mm/d or 3.5 cm/wk. At approximately 5 to 6 weeks, a yolk sac/embryo complex can be seen within the chorionic sac (Fig. 7-3). The embryo can be identified as a echogenic focus immediately adjacent to a pole of the yolk sac. When the embryo measures 5 mm or more, heart motion can consistently be identified, but only if scanners with high frame rate (over 30 frames/sec) are used (Fig. 7-4). A recent study has shown that normal embryos less than 4 mm may not demonstrate heart motion and follow-up examination of these embryos is warranted (Levi et al, 1990). Measurement of the crown–rump length of the embryo with TVS provides an accurate determination of gestational age (Degenhardt et al, 1988) (Table 7-2).

TVS Features

The chorionic sac can be seen in most intrauterine pregnancies when β-human chorionic gonadotropin (β-hCG) level is above 500 mIU/mL (2nd International Standard) (Bree et al, 1989) (Table 7-3). This is particularly important when examining a patient in whom there is a clinical suspicion of ectopic pregnancy (Fleischer et al, 1990).

Punctate hypoechoic areas representing blood pools or vascular lacunae can be seen surrounding the developing chorion (Fig. 7-5). When these are large (approximating the size of the gestational sac) and hypoechoic, they are called retrochorionic hemorrhage (Fig. 7-6). As documented in one study, these hemorrhages are usually associated with a good prognosis for completion of pregnancy (Stabile et al, 1989). If they are over one-fourth of the volume of the gestational sac size, they may be associated with spontaneous abortion. Follow-up sonography is recommended in these patients.

The embryo is seen consistently when it measures over 5 mm, which corresponds to approximately 5 to 6 weeks gestational age. Heart contractions begin at this time and usually can be estimated to be above 80 to 90 beats/min (DuBose et al, 1988). This rate occurs when the heart is forming; there is a slow increase in heart rate up to approximately 10 weeks in size, when the heart rate is usually between 140- and 180 beats/min (Hertzberg et al, 1988).

Certain anatomic features of the embryo/fetus can be seen in detail with TVS. Similarly, some of the normal developmental features delineated by TVS may be mistaken for abnormal. For example, an extra yolk sac or allantoic cysts of the developing umbilical cord may be seen in early fetal development and require follow-up scans (Barzilai et al, 1989) (Fig. 7-7). The rhombencephalon appears as a hypoechoic area within

Table 7-1   TVS "Landmarks"

Gestational Age	Sign
4 wks	Choriodecidual thickening; chorionic sac
5 wks	Chorionic sac (5 to 15 mm); yolk sac
6 wks	Yolk sac/embryo; detectable heart motion
7 wks	Embryo/fetal movement; prominent rhombencephalon
8 wks	Physiologic bowel herniation; arms, legs

the posterior aspect of the fetal head corresponding to developing of the fourth ventricle and posterior fossa structures and should not be confused with yolk sac, which is extra-amniotic (Fig. 7-8). Physiologic herniation of the bowel into the base of the umbilical cord can be identified at 8 to 9 weeks, but should spontaneously regress by 12 weeks (Fig. 7-9).

From 8 weeks on, several anatomic structures of the developing fetus can be delineated in detail with TVS. These include the arms and hands, legs and the facial structures, the ventricular system and choroid plexus, as well as the spine (Fig. 7-10). Extrafetal structures that can be seen include the amnion, which appears as a thin membrane surrounding the fetus. It separates the amniotic cavity from the extraembryonic coelom. Fetal body activity can be identified as early

as 6 to 8 weeks and usually consists of flexion or extension of the fetal body and movement of the fetal extremities.

The improved resolution of fetal structures by TVS allows the diagnosis of some fetal gross anomalies such as anencephaly in the first trimester. The problem of misdiagnosis as abnormal of an unusual feature during embryonic/fetal development also exists, however.

Tables 7-4 to 7-7 contain data concerning embryonic and fetal biometry during the first trimester (Timor-Tritsch et al, 1990).

Twin Pregnancy

Twin pregnancy can accurately be identified as early as 5 to 6 weeks after conception by the presence of more than one chorionic sac. Dichorionic placental development can be predicted if the two sacs are separate from each other (Fig. 7-11). Similarly, the amnionicity of twin pregnancies can be seen during the first trimester by establishment of the continuity of the amnion surrounding each fetus (Fig. 7-12).

Summary

The role of TVS in early pregnancy is to confirm the presence of an intrauterine pregnancy or to provide

Table 7-2   CRL Versus Gestational Age (wks)

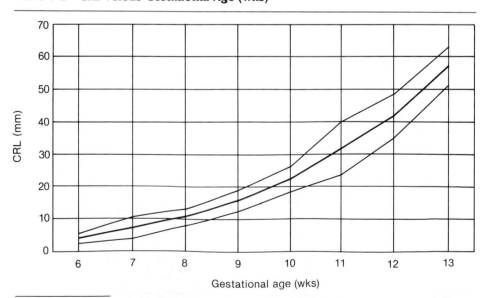

From Degenhardt F, Böhmer S, Behrens O, Mühlhaus K: Transvaginale Ultraschallbiometrie der Scheitel-Steiss-Länge im ersten Trimenon. *Z Geburtshilfe Perinatol* 1988;192:249–252.

Table 7-3   TVS "Milestones" Versus β-hCG

	β-hCG	d	wks
Gestational sac	1000 mIU/mL (IRP)	32	4+
Yolk sac	7200 mIU/mL (IRP)	36 to 40	5 to 6
Embryo with heart motion	10800 mIU/mL (IRP)	<40	6+

IRP, international reference preparation.

From Bree RL, Edwards M, Bohm-Velez M, Beyler S, Roberts J, Mendelson EB: Transvaginal sonography in the evaluation of normal early pregnancy: Correlation with HCG level. *AJR* 1989;153:75–79.

Table 7-4   Gestational Age Versus Crown–Rump Length (cm)

Gestational Age (wks)	5th Percentile	50th Percentile	95th Percentile
6	0.15	0.28	0.47
7	0.47	0.70	1.03
8	0.95	1.32	1.82
9	1.61	2.13	2.83
10	2.43	3.14	4.07
11	3.43	4.34	5.52
12	4.60	5.74	7.20
13	5.94	7.33	9.10
14	7.44	9.11	11.22

From Timor-Tritsch I, Lassen D, Peisner D, et al: Embryonic and fetal biometry in the first trimester as depicted with TVS. *J Ultrasound Med* 1990;9(suppl):S41.

Table 7-6   Gestational Age Versus Head Circumference (cm)

Gestational Age (wks)	5th Percentile	50th Percentile	95th Percentile
9	2.05	3.20	4.78
10	3.23	4.57	6.35
11	4.42	5.91	7.92
12	5.59	7.26	9.49
13	6.78	8.61	11.06
14	7.96	9.95	12.63

From Timor-Tritsch I, Lassen D, Peisner D, et al: Embryonic and fetal biometry in the first trimester as depicted with TVS. *J Ultrasound Med* 1990;9(suppl):S41.

Table 7-5   Gestational Age Versus Biparietal Diameter (cm)

Gestational Age (wks)	5th Percentile	50th Percentile	95th Percentile
7	0.46	0.47	0.48
8	0.62	0.63	0.64
9	0.82	0.86	0.91
10	1.07	1.16	1.28
11	1.40	1.56	1.82
12	1.83	2.11	2.57
13	2.37	2.85	3.64
14	3.08	3.85	5.15

From Timor-Tritsch I, Lassen D, Peisner D, et al: Embryonic and fetal biometry in the first trimester as depicted with TVS. *J Ultrasound Med* 1990;9(suppl):S41.

Table 7-7   Gestational Age Versus Abdominal Circumference (cm)

Gestational Age (wks)	5th Percentile	50th Percentile	95th Percentile
9	1.89	2.85	3.16
10	2.32	3.62	6.95
11	2.85	4.62	9.36
12	3.49	5.88	12.61
13	4.28	7.59	16.98

From Timor-Tritsch I, Lassen D, Peisner D, et al: Embryonic and fetal biometry in the first trimester as depicted with TVS. *J Ultrasound Med* 1990;9(suppl):S41.

definitive diagnosis of an ectopic pregnancy by demonstration of an adnexal mass and no intrauterine gestational sac (Fleischer, 1990). TVS should be carefully applied, and misdiagnosis due to lack of experience with unusual development anatomy should be avoided by adopting a conservative approach.

References

Barzilai M, Lyons EA, Levi CS, Lindsay DJ. Vitelline duct cyst or double yolk sac. *J Ultrasound Med* 1989;8:523–526.

Bree RL, Edwards M, Bohm-Velez M, Beyler S, Roberts J, Mendelson EB. Transvaginal sonography in the evaluation of normal early pregnancy: correlation with HCG level. *AJR* 1989;153:75–79.

Cyr DR, Mack LA, Nyberg DA, Shepard TH, Shuman WP. Fetal rhombencephalon: normal US findings. *Radiology* 166:691–692.

de Crespigny L, Cooper D, McKenna M. Early detection of intrauterine pregnancy with ultrasound. *J Ultrasound Med* 1988;7:7–10.

Degenhardt F, Böhmer S, Behrens O, Mühlhaus K. Transvaginale Ultraschallbiometrie der Scheitel-Steiss-Länge im ersten Trimenon. *Z Geburtshilfe Perinatol* 1988;192:249–252.

DuBose TJ, Dickey D, Butschek CM, Porter L, Hill LW, Poole EK. The opinion that the fetal heart rate (FHR) is an indicator of the baby's sex (letter). *J Ultrasound Med* 1988;7:237–238.

Fleischer AC, Pennell RG, McKee MS, et al. Sonographic features of ectopic pregnancies as depicted by transvaginal scanning. *Radiology* 1990;174:375–378.

Hertzberg BS, Mahony BS, Bowie JD. First trimester fetal cardiac activity: sonographic documentation of a progressive early rise in heart rate. *J Ultrasound Med* 1988;7:573–575.

Jain KA, Hamper UM, Sanders RC. Comparison of transvaginal and transabdominal sonography in the detection of early pregnancy and its complications. *AJR* 1988;151:1139–1143.

Levi CS, Lyons EA, Lindsay DJ. Early diagnosis of nonviable pregnancy with endovaginal US. *Radiology* 1988;167:383–385.

Levi CS, Lyons EA, Zheng XH, Lindsay DJ, Holt SC. Endovaginal US demonstration of cardiac activity in embryos of less than 5.0 mm in crown-rump length. *Radiology* 1990;176:71–74.

Pennell RG, Baltarowich OH, Kurtz AB, et al: Complicated first-trimester pregnancies: evaluation with endovaginal US versus transabdominal technique. *Radiology* 1987;165:79–83.

Stabile I, Campbell S, Grudzinskas JG. Threatened miscarriage and intrauterine hematomas: sonographic and biochemical studies. *J Ultrasound Med* 1989;8:289–292.

Timor-Tritsch IE, Lasser D, Peisner D, Vollebergh J. Embryonic and fetal biometry in the first trimester as depicted with TVS. *J Ultrasound Med* 1990;9(suppl) 41.

FIGURE 7-1   Thickened Decidua at 2 5/7 Weeks After a Successful IVF-ER Procedure

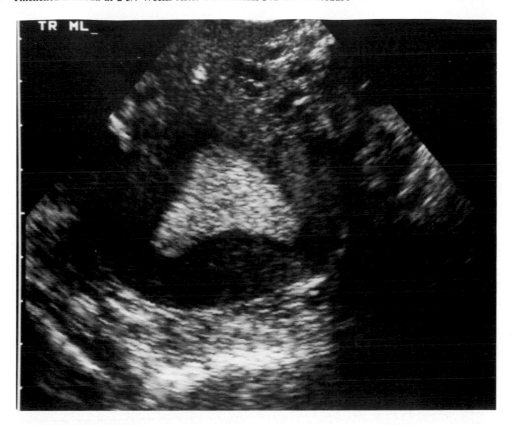

DECIDUALIZED ENDOMETRIUM

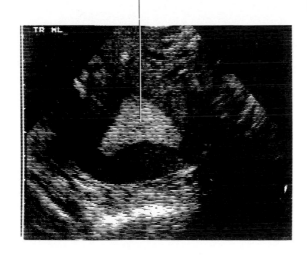

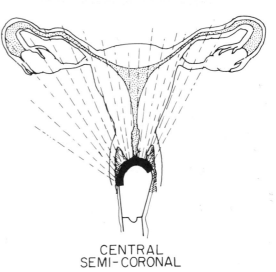

CENTRAL
SEMI-CORONAL

FIGURE 7-2 Chorionic Sac within Thickened Choriodecidua of 4-Week Intrauterine Pregnancy

7-2A Chorionic sac with decidualized endometrium at 4 weeks.

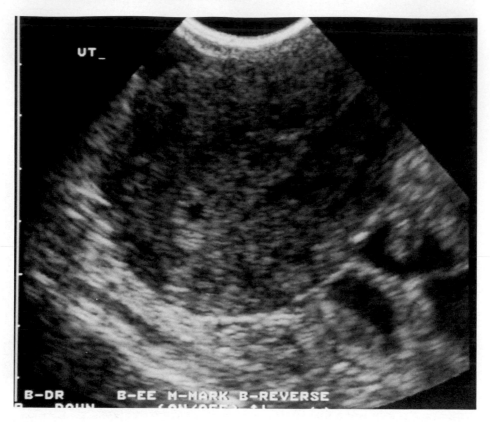

CHORIONIC SAC

DECIDUA

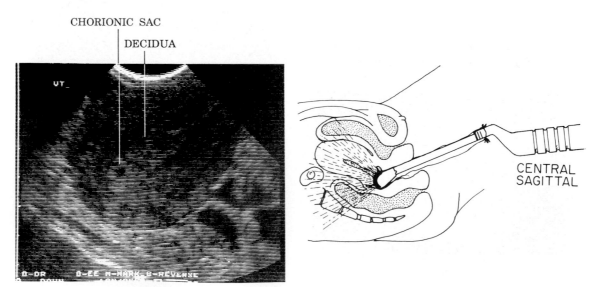

CENTRAL
SAGITTAL

FIGURE 7-2   Chorionic Sac within Thickened Choriodecidua of 4-Week Intrauterine Pregnancy *(continued)*

7-2B   Chorionic sac within thickened choriodecidua in 5-week intrauterine pregnancy.
β-hCG = 1500 mIU/mL (2nd Int. St.).

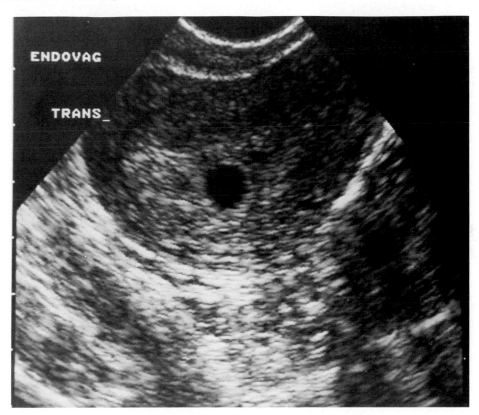

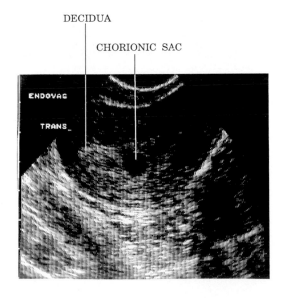

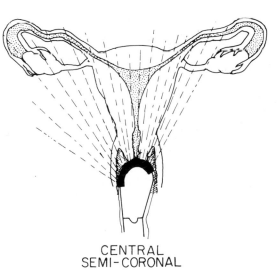

FIGURE 7-3   Four- to Five-Week Intrauterine Pregnancy

7-3A   Chorionic sac with developing yolk sac.

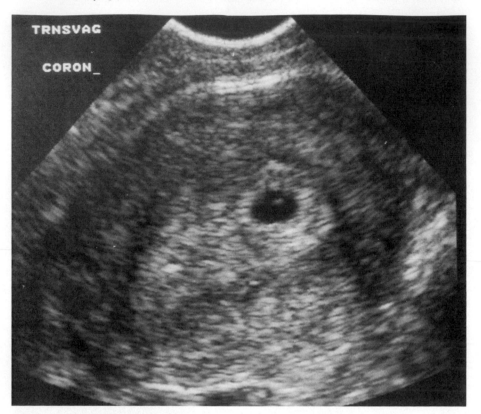

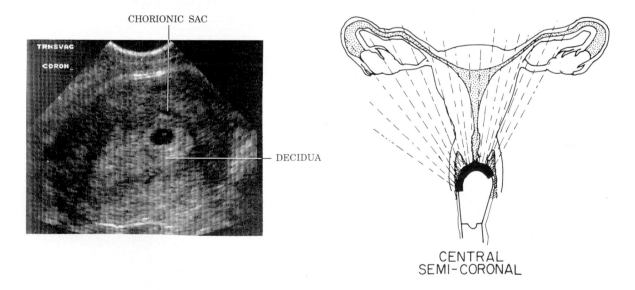

CHORIONIC SAC

DECIDUA

CENTRAL
SEMI-CORONAL

FIGURE 7-3   **Four- to Five-Week Intrauterine Pregnancy** *(continued)*

7-3B   Chorionic sac with developing yolk sac/embryo.

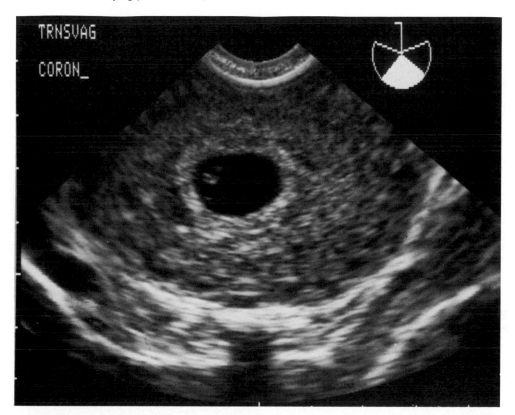

YOLK SAC/ EMBRYO

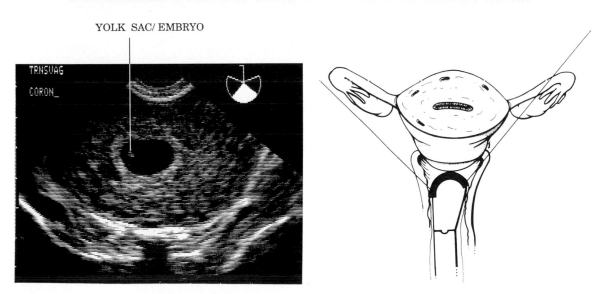

(continued)

FIGURE 7-3   Four- to Five-Week Intrauterine Pregnancy *(continued)*

7-3C   Yolk sac/embryo/amniotic sac forming a "double bleb." This formation is present for 1 or 2 days only.

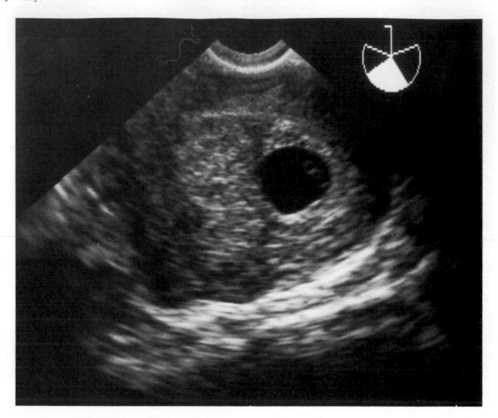

YOLK SAC/ EMBRYO

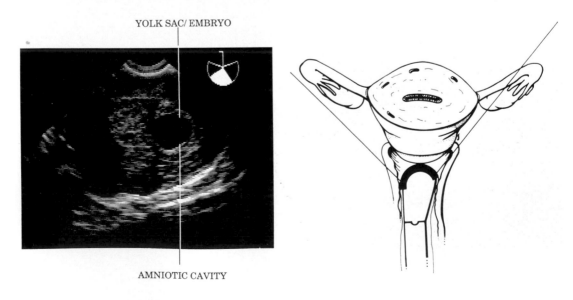

AMNIOTIC CAVITY

FIGURE 7-3   Four- to Five-Week Intrauterine Pregnancy *(continued)*

7-3D   Yolk sac/embryo within gestational sac.

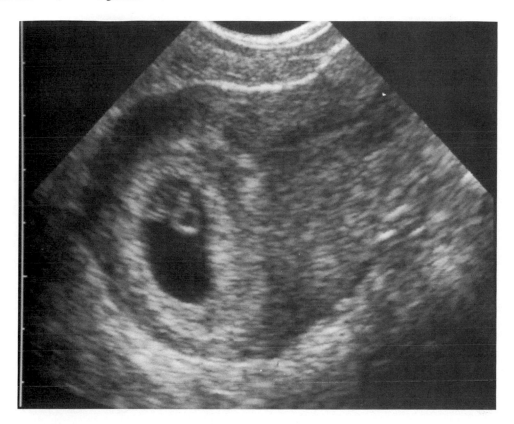

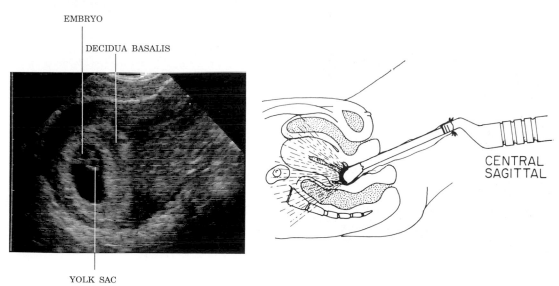

EMBRYO

DECIDUA BASALIS

YOLK SAC

CENTRAL SAGITTAL

FIGURE 7-4   Six- to Seven-Week Intrauterine Pregnancy

7-4A   Magnified scan of 4-mm embryo within inferior aspect of gestational sac.

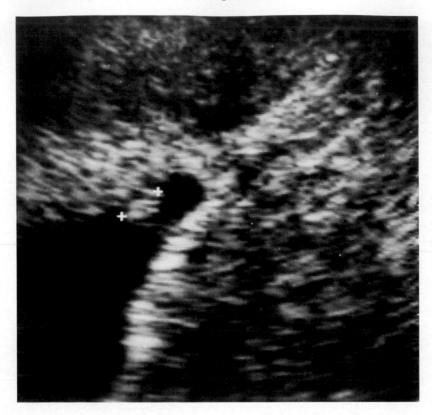

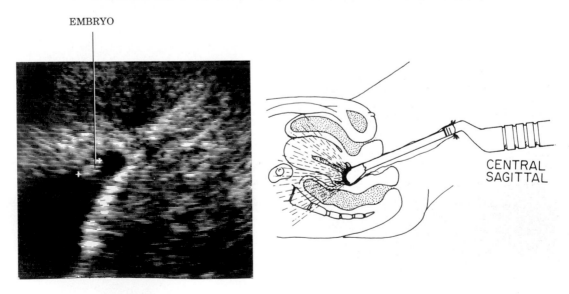

EMBRYO

CENTRAL
SAGITTAL

FIGURE 7-4   Six- to Seven-Week Intrauterine Pregnancy *(continued)*

7-4B   Developing spine and spinal cord in 6-week embryo. The yolk sac is adjacent to the embryo.

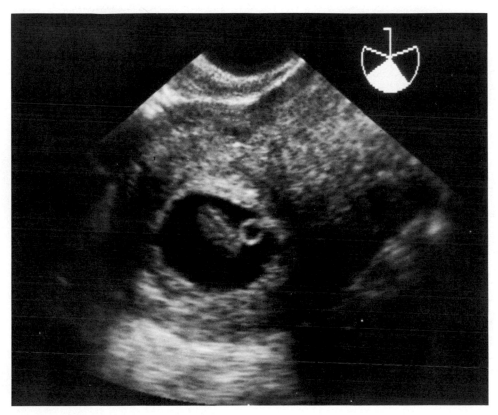

DEVELOPING SPINE

(continued)

FIGURE 7-4   Six- to Seven-Week Intrauterine Pregnancy *(continued)*

7-4C   Heart motion depicted in M-mode of a 7-week embryo.

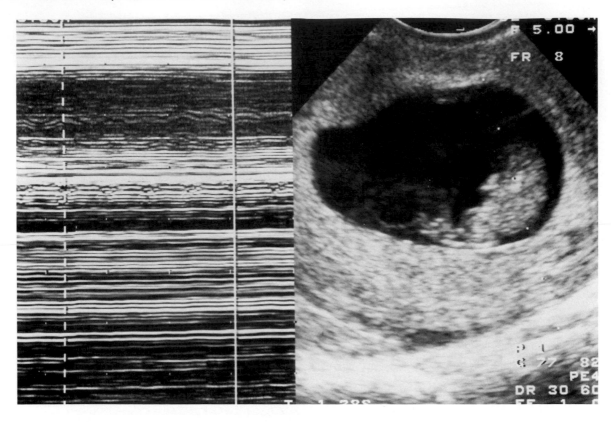

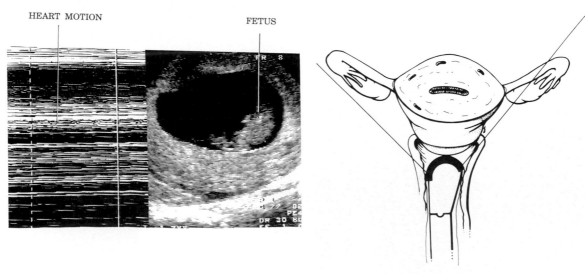

FIGURE 7-5   Normal Variants

7-5A   Vascular lacunae behind decidua basalis.

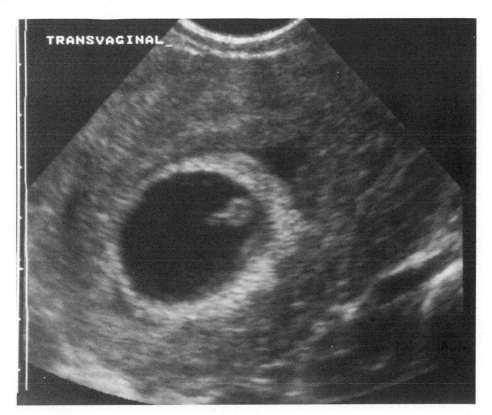

DECIDUA BASALIS

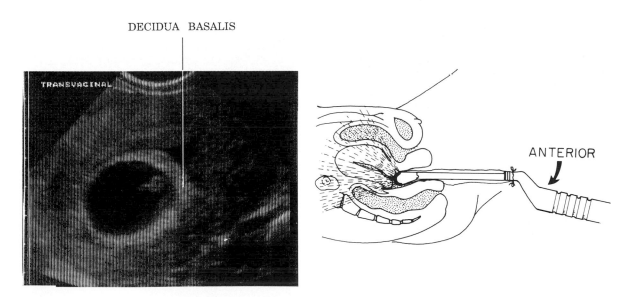

ANTERIOR

(continued)

FIGURE 7-5   **Normal Variants** *(continued)*

7-5B   Corpus luteum cysts with 6-week intrauterine pregnancy.

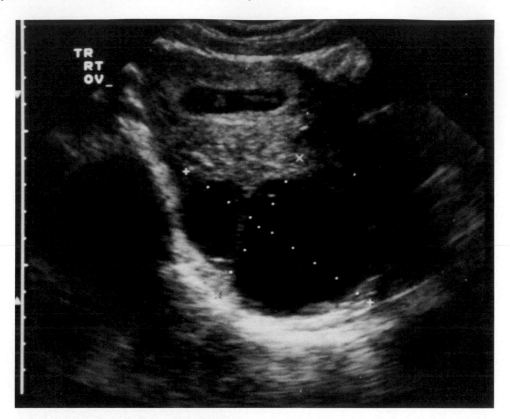

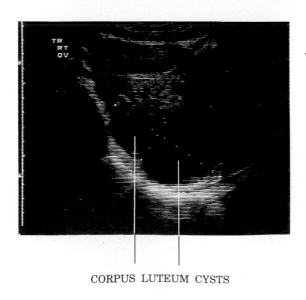

CORPUS LUTEUM CYSTS

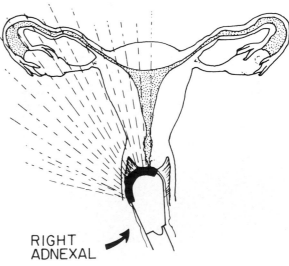

RIGHT
ADNEXAL

FIGURE 7-5   Normal Variants *(continued)*

7-5C   Bicornuate uterus with 7-week intrauterine pregnancy in left horn and decidualized endometrium in right horn.

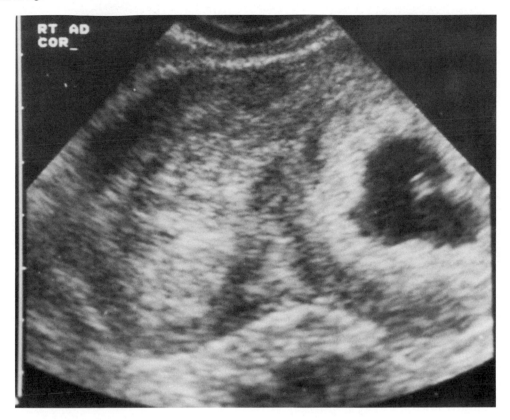

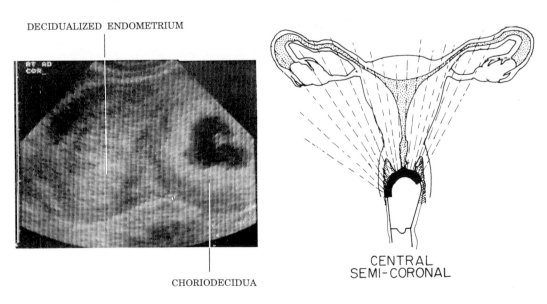

DECIDUALIZED ENDOMETRIUM

CHORIODECIDUA

CENTRAL
SEMI-CORONAL

FIGURE 7-6   Retrochorionic Hemorrhage Appearing as Hypoechoic Area Adjacent to Gestational Sac

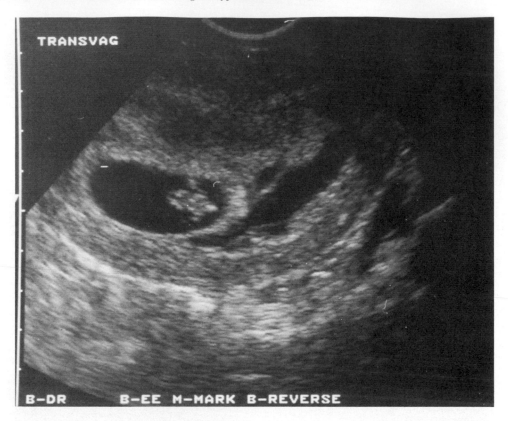

RETROCHORIONIC HEMORRHAGE

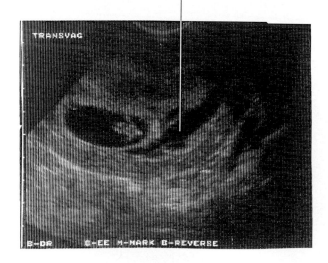

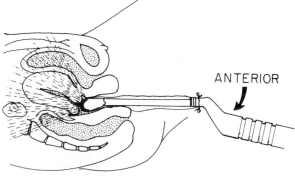

FIGURE 7-7   Eight-Week Fetus with Physiologic Bowel Herniation and an Allantoic Cyst Contiguous within the Developing Umbilical Cord

7-7A   Long-axis.

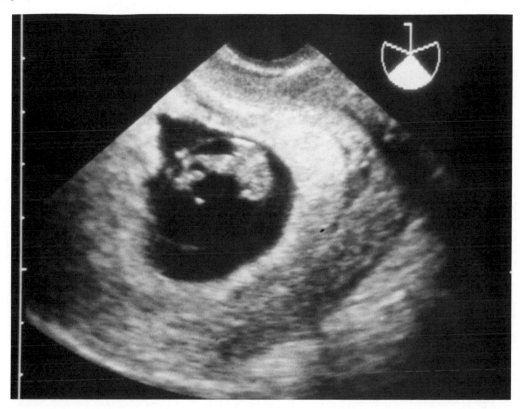

PHYSIOLOGICAL BOWEL HERNIATION

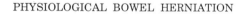

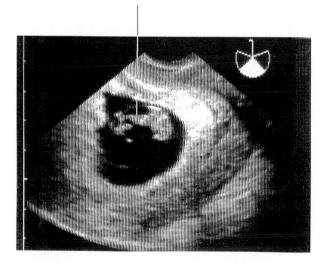

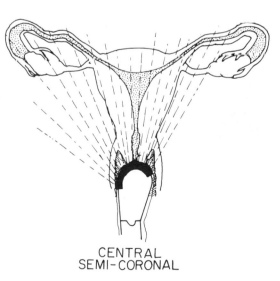

CENTRAL
SEMI-CORONAL

(continued)

FIGURE 7-7   Eight-Week Fetus with Physiologic Bowel Herniation and an Allantoic Cyst Contiguous within the Developing Umbilical Cord *(continued)*

7-7B   Short-axis.

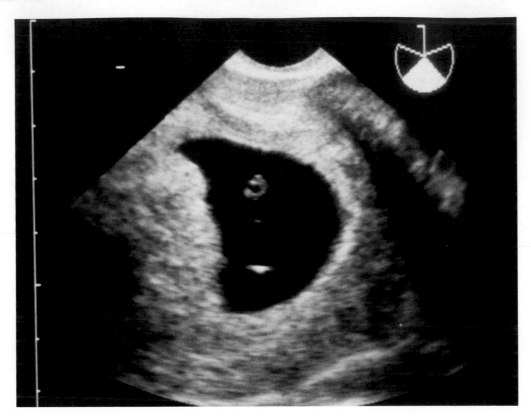

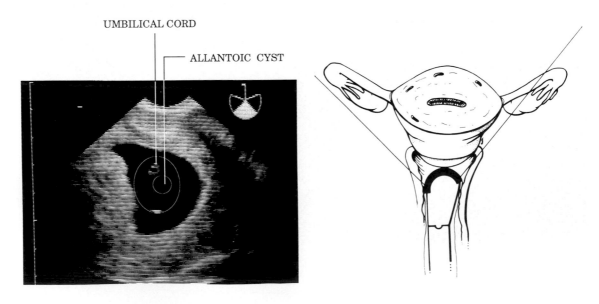

FIGURE 7-8   Cystic Area in Posterior Portion of Cranium in 7-Week Embryo Representing the Rhombencephalon

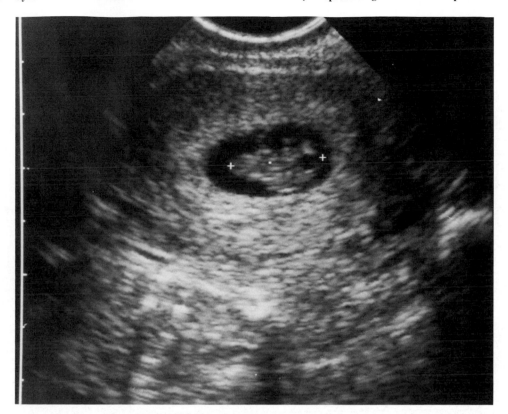

RHOMBENCEPHALON

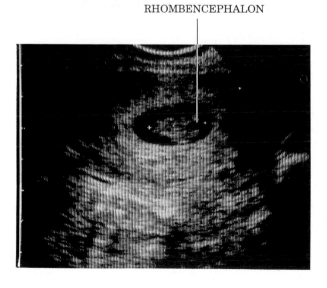

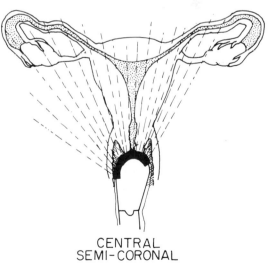

CENTRAL
SEMI-CORONAL

FIGURE 7-9   Physiologic Bowel Herniation

7-9A   Physiologic bowel herniation into base of umbilical cord at 9 weeks.

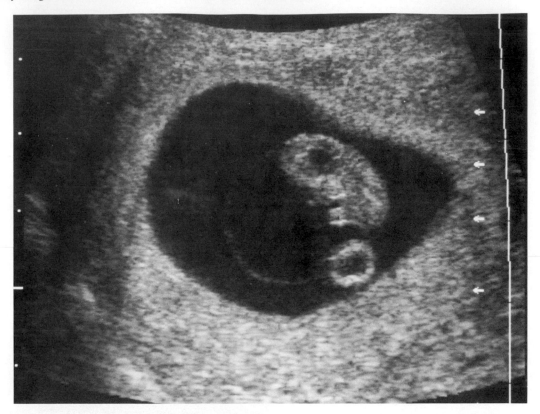

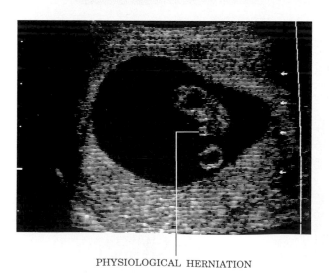

PHYSIOLOGICAL HERNIATION

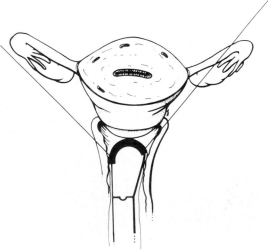

FIGURE 7-9   Physiologic Bowel Herniation *(continued)*

7-9B   More prominent herniation in a 9-week fetus. This prompted a repeat scan at 12 weeks that showed return of bowel contents into the abdomen.

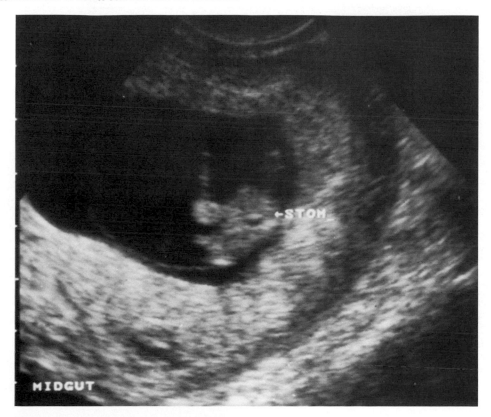

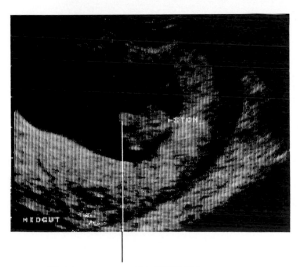

PHYSIOLOGIC HERNIATION

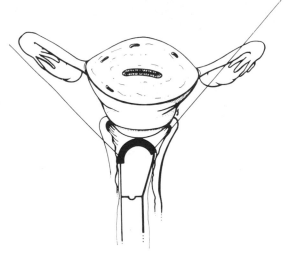

FIGURE 7-10   Normal 10-Week Fetus and Membranes

7-10A   Normal lateral ventricles and choroid plexus in 10-week fetus.

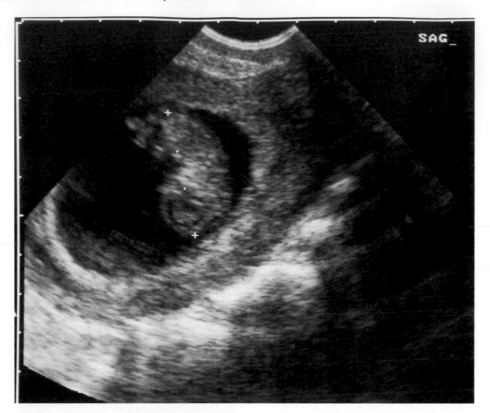

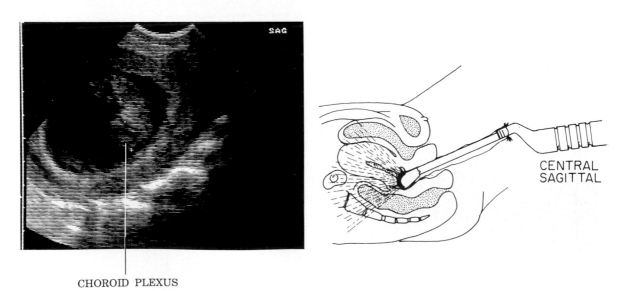

CHOROID PLEXUS

CENTRAL
SAGITTAL

FIGURE 7-10   Normal 10-Week Fetus and Membranes *(continued)*

7-10B   Normal 10-week fetus in long-axis view.

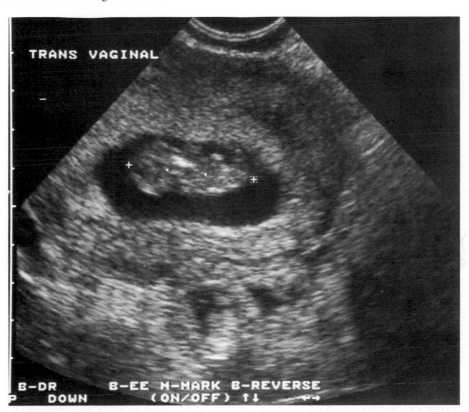

FETUS

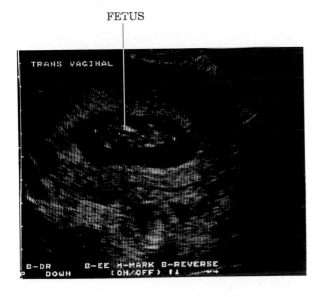

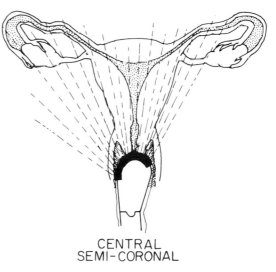

CENTRAL
SEMI-CORONAL

(continued)

FIGURE 7-10   Normal 10-Week Fetus and Membranes *(continued)*

7-10C   Normal arms and legs of a 10-week fetus. The amnion is seen as a thin interface surrounding the fetus.

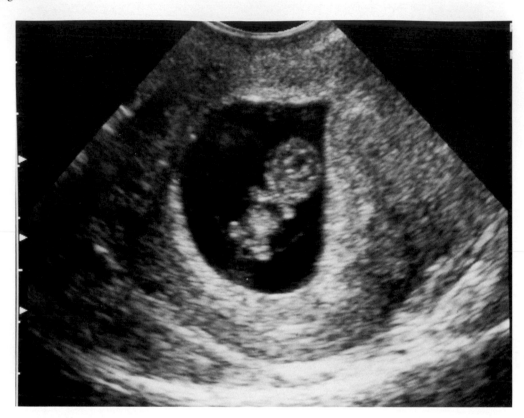

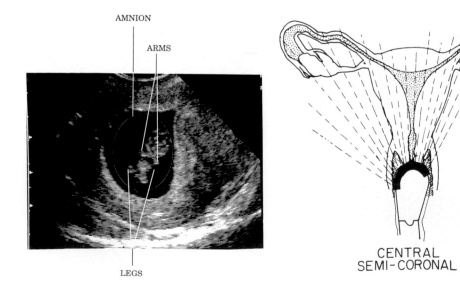

FIGURE 7-10   Normal 10-Week Fetus and Membranes *(continued)*

7-10D   Normal 9-week fetus within amniotic cavity.

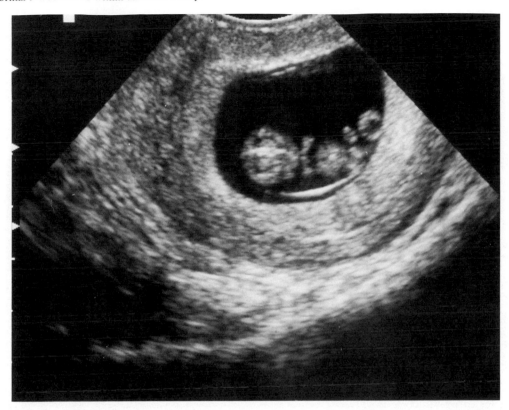

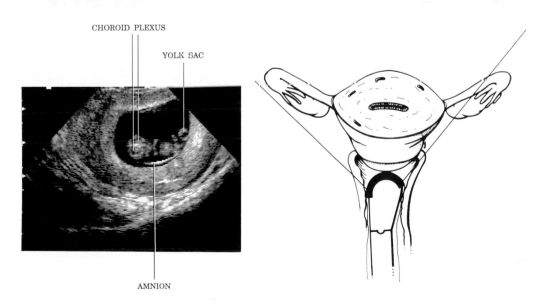

CHOROID PLEXUS

YOLK SAC

AMNION

(continued)

FIGURE 7-10   **Normal 10-Week Fetus and Membranes** *(continued)*

7-10E   Normal cerebellum in 11-week fetus.

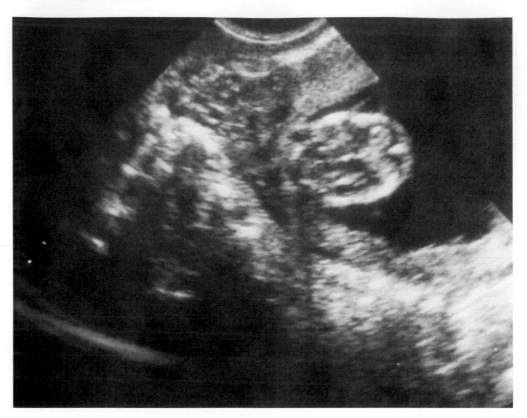

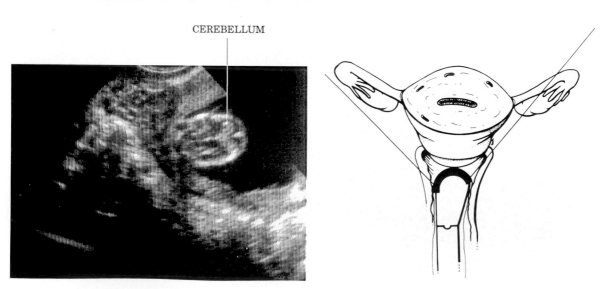

CEREBELLUM

FIGURE 7-10   Normal 10-Week Fetus and Membranes *(continued)*

7-10F   Normal developing spine of a 10-week fetus.

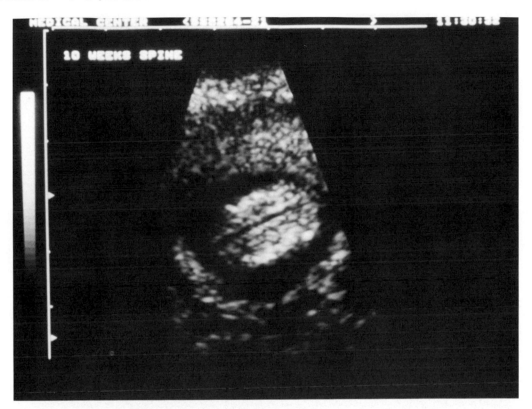

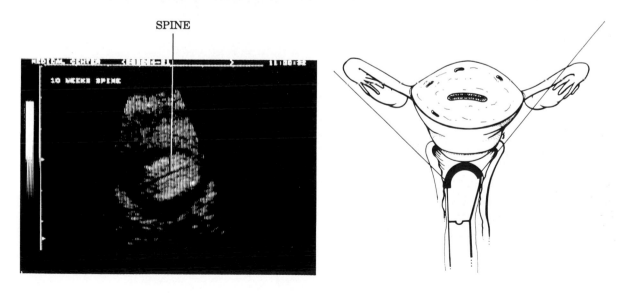

FIGURE 7-11   Normal Diamniotic Twin Intrauterine Pregnancy

7-11A   Twin separate (dizygotic) sacs at 5 weeks.

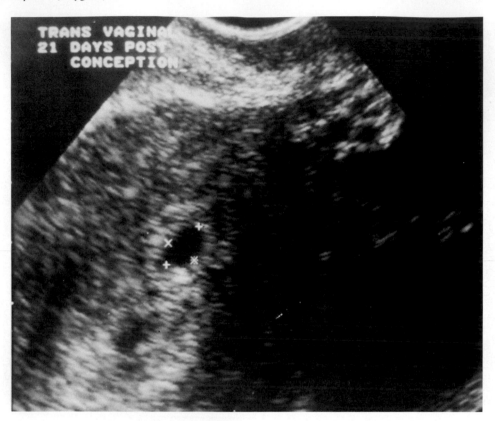

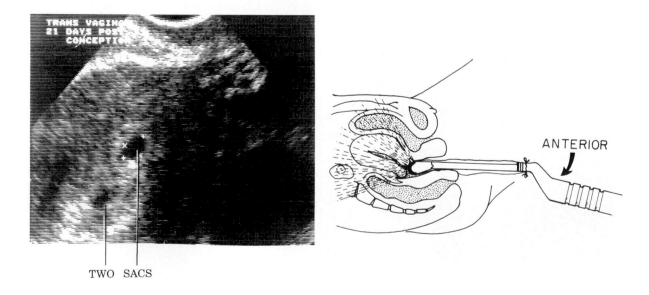

TWO   SACS

FIGURE 7-11   Normal Diamniotic Twin Intrauterine Pregnancy *(continued)*

7-11B   Diamniotic twin intrauterine pregnancy at 7 weeks.

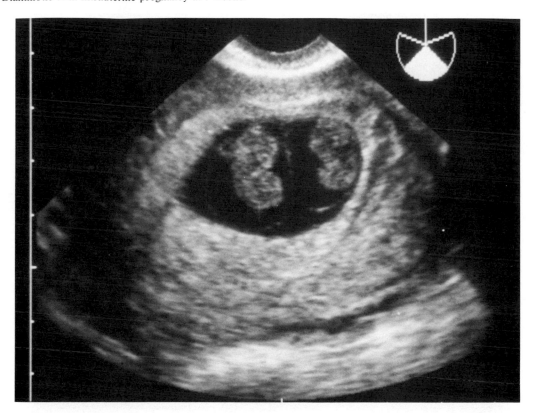

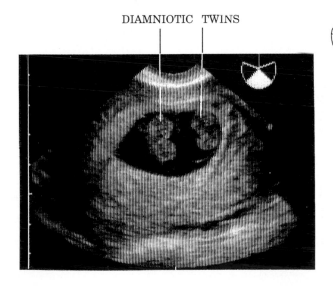

DIAMNIOTIC TWINS

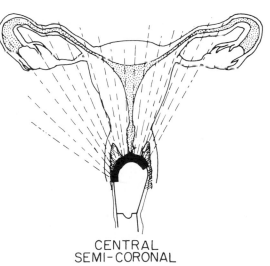

CENTRAL
SEMI-CORONAL

FIGURE 7-12   Monoamniotic Twin Intrauterine Pregnancy

7-12A   6-week monoamniotic twins.

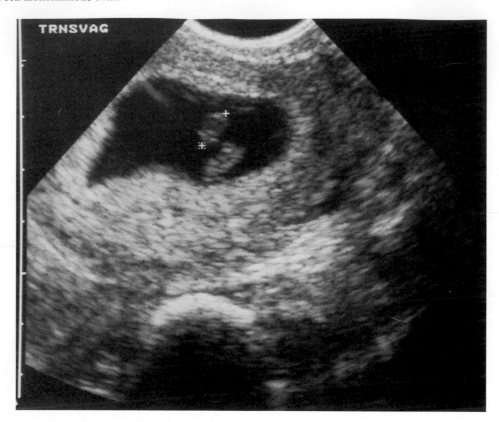

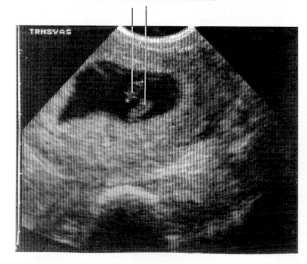

MONOAMNIOTIC TWINS

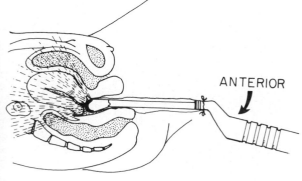

ANTERIOR

FIGURE 7-12   Monoamniotic Twin Intrauterine Pregnancy *(continued)*

7-12B   Demise of both twins at 8 weeks.

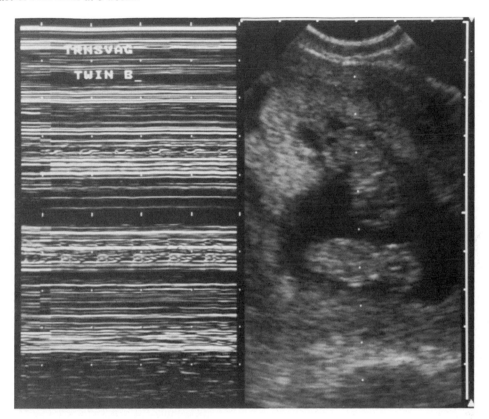

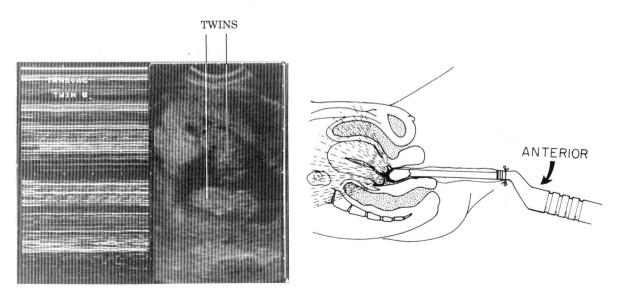

Chapter 8

Complicated Early Pregnancy

Arthur C. Fleischer, MD
Donna M. Kepple, RDMS

Introduction

Transvaginal sonography (TVS) depicts detailed anatomic structures and reveals some functional aspects of early pregnancies, such as heart and body motion. The assessment of a complicated pregnancy obtained by TVS provides important clinical information so that the patient can be optimally managed. Specifically, TVS reveals important information concerning the presence or absence of an embryo/fetus and whether there is heart motion, the intactness of the choriodecidua, and the location (intrauterine or extrauterine) of the gestation.

Embryonic/Fetal Demise

In a normal pregnancy, heart motion should be demonstrated by TVS in embryos that are over 5 mm or 5 to 6 weeks gestation. The actual rate is relatively slow during early heart development (70 to 90 beats/min) but increases at approximately 8 weeks to approximately 120 beats/min (DuBose, 1989; Hertzberg et al, 1988). Some authors have observed that embryos between 6 and 9 weeks with slow heart rates (less than 85 beats/min) have a tendency to spontaneously abort (Laboda et al, 1989). The embryo with a slow heart rate should always be given the benefit of the doubt, however, and be reexamined in 3 to 5 days for signs of conversion back to a normal heart rate.

Early embryonic demise has a variety of appearances, ranging from a gestational sac devoid of a yolk sac or embryo to a yolk sac–embryo complex without embryonic heart motion (Fig. 8-1). Embryonic demise should be suspected when there is a lack of enlargement of the embryo on serial scan coupled with deflation of the sac or yolk sac. In some cases of embryonic demise, there is deflation of the yolk sac coupled with an increase in its internal echogenicity.

One should not terminate the pregnancy based on a single sonographic examination that demonstrates a lack of heart motion during the embryonic stage (3 to 5 mm crown rump length [CRL]) of development. A follow-up scan is usually indicated to confirm the lack of embryonic or fetal viability. In general, an embryo should be seen in a sac larger than 6 to 9 mm; embryonic heart motion should be seen when the sac is 10 to 14 mm in size (Bree et al, 1989).

Embryonic loss is believed to occur in approximately 20% to 30% of all developing early pregnancies (Biggers, 1982). It is more likely in the patient with a history of abortion (habitual aborter) or a previous fetus with chromosomal abnormality.

Abortion

Incomplete spontaneous abortion demonstrates echogenic tissue within the uterine lumen arising from retained choriodecidua (Fig. 8-2A). Completed abortion may be diagnosed occasionally when there is no echogenic tissue (decidualized endometrium or blood) within the uterine lumen and when the cervical os is closed (Fig. 8-2D). The relative amount of remaining choriodecidua can be estimated using a prolate ellipsoid formula

$$\text{vol in cc} = \text{length [cm]} \times \text{height [cm]} \times \text{width [cm]} \times 0.5$$

Early trophoblastic disease demonstrates a pattern similar to retained choriodecidua, and hydropic villi are usually not present before 14 weeks (Fig. 8-3A).

Patients who experience vaginal bleeding in the first trimester may demonstrate areas of retrochorionic hemorrhage on TVS. Retrochorionic hemorrhage appears as relatively hypoechoic areas behind the chorionic layer. If it is small and remote to the decidua basalis, the chance for pregnancy completion is better than if it extends behind the decidua basalis or is over 25% of the size of the gestational sac (Sauerbrei and Pham, 1986) (Fig. 8-3*B*).

Ectopic Pregnancy

TVS is an accurate means of diagnosing an ectopic pregnancy (Nyberg et al, 1987; Dafechesky et al, 1988, Fleischer et al, 1990). First, an intrauterine gestational sac can be excluded earlier (1 to 2 weeks) with TVS than with transabdominal scanning. Second, the ability to detect the adnexal mass that represents an ectopic pregnancy is significantly enhanced with TVS.

Intraluminal fluid or blood surrounding the thin decidua reaction in an ectopic pregnancy occasionally stimulates the appearance of a malformed gestational sac. The thickened decidual reaction that surrounds intraluminal fluid or blood (''pseudosac'') seen in some advanced ectopic pregnancies can be distinguished from a normal gestational sac because the choriodecidual thickening at the decidua basalis is not present (Fig. 8-4).

In the adnexa, TVS demonstrates the presence of a ''tubal ring'' consisting of an echogenic rim and a hypoechoic center (Fig. 8-5). This structure is typically seen in the adnexal regions adjacent to but separate from the uterus and ovary. An embryo may or may not be seen within the gestational sac, since a large number of ectopic gestations have chromosomal abnormalities with resultant embryonic demise and fail to develop a sonographically detectable embryo. One can usually distinguish the tubal ring from a corpus luteum because the corpus luteum is located within the displaced rim of ovarian tissue. In some patients with a centrally located corpus luteum, the TVS appearance of a tubal ring was mimicked. Some corpora lutea appear as hypoechoic masses that have broken linear interfaces within probably representing synechiae. Most hematomas associated with ectopic pregnancy appear as solid rounded masses that displace the uterus and bowel out of the cul-de-sac. In unruptured tubal ectopic pregnancies, the tubal ring is distinct. The distended tube surrounding the tubal mass may be identified.

If rupture has occurred, the fallopian tube is enlarged, fusiform and contains irregularly echogenic material. Intraperitoneal blood may be the result of blood oozing from the fimbriated end of the tube because of detachment of the chorionic tissue from the tubal wall (Fig. 8-6). It may also result from attempts at tubal abortion, where the gestational sac is passed out through the fimbriated end of the tube. The intraperitoneal fluid associated with a ruptured ectopic pregnancy usually has echoes within it, reflecting a predominance of clotted blood rather than serous fluid. The low-level echoes arising from blood elements suspended within intraperitoneal fluid move in a swirling pattern when the bowel peristalses around them.

Unusual types of ectopic pregnancy can be recognized with TVS. These include cornual, cervical, and ovarian ectopic pregnancies. Cornual ectopic pregnancy form eccenteric to the endometrial lumen and extend to within 3 to 5 mm of the uterine serosa. Hypoechoic blood lacunae may be seen surrounding the gestation. Cervical ectopic pregnancies form proximal to the endometrial tissue and distend the cervix. They can be distinguished from cervical inclusion cysts by the relatively thick choriodecidual layer that surrounds the hypoechoic lumen (Fig. 8-7). This appearance is similar to choriodecidua in the process of being aborted except that cervical ectopic pregnancies are usually better defined and remote from the endometrial lumen. Ovarian ectopic pregnancies are extremely rare. The examples that have been seen appear as hypoechoic areas within the ovary when a solid component of an embryo is present.

Summary

TVS has an important role in the evaluation of a complicated early pregnancy. Specifically, incomplete abortion, embryonic demise, and ectopic pregnancy are readily diagnosed with this method.

References

Biggers S. In vitro fertilization and embryo transfer in human beings. *N Engl J Med* 1982;304:336–342.

Bree RL, Edwards M, Bohm-Velez M, Beyler S, Roberts J, Mendelson EB. Transvaginal sonography in the evaluation of normal early pregnancy: correlation with HCG level. *AJR* 1989;153:75–79.

Dashefsky SM, Lyons EA, Levi CS, Lindsay DJ. Suspected ectopic pregnancy: endovaginal and transvesical US. *Radiology* 1988;169:181–184.

DuBose T. Fetal heart rates. *J Ultrasound Med* 1989;8:407–408. Letter to the Editor.

Fleischer AC, Pennell RG, McKee MS, et al. Sonographic features of ectopic pregnancies as depicted by transvaginal scanning. *Radiology* 1990;174:375–378.

Hertzberg BS, Mahony BS, Bowie JD. First trimester fetal cardiac activity: sonographic documentation of a progressive early rise in heart rate. *J Ultrasound Med* 1988;7:573–575.

Laboda LA, Estroff JA, Benacerraf BR. First trimester brady-cardia. *J Ultrasound Med* 1989;8:561–563.

Levi CS, Lyons EA, Lindsay DJ. Early diagnosis of nonviable pregnancy with endovaginal US. *Radiology* 1988;167:383–385.

Nyberg DA, Mack LA, Jeffrey RB, Laing FC. Endovaginal sonographic evaluation of ectopic pregnancy: a prospective study. *AJR* 1987;149:1181–1186.

Pennell RG, Baltarowich OH, Kurtz AB, et al. Complicated first-trimester pregnancies: evaluation with endovaginal US versus transabdominal technique. *Radiology* 1987;165:79–83.

Sauerbrei, EE, Pham DH. Placental abruption and subchorionic hemorrhage in the first half of pregnancy: US appearance and clinical outcome. *Radiology* 1986;160:109–112.

FIGURE 8-1 Embryonic Demise

8-1A Initial TVS showing yolk sac within the gestational sac.

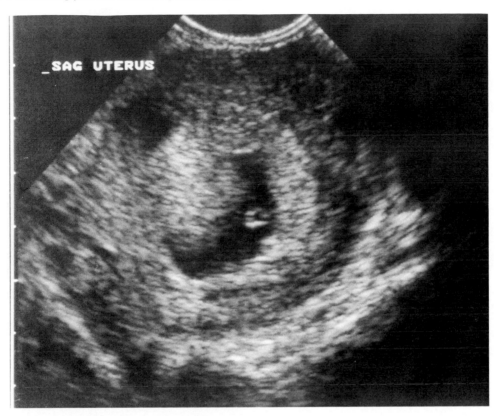

YOLK SAC

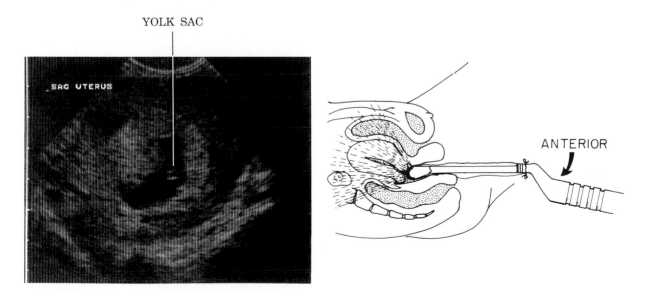

(continued)

FIGURE 8-1   **Embryonic Demise** *(continued)*

8-1B   Three days later there has been deflation of the gestational sac.

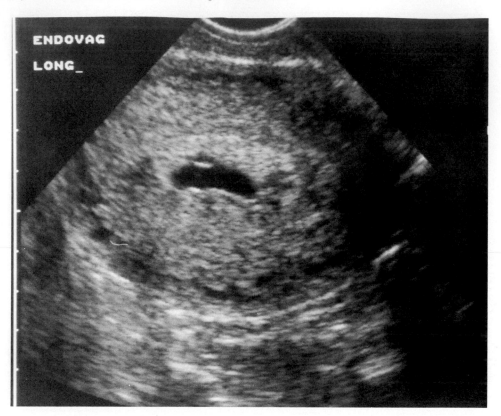

"DEFLATED" SAC

FIGURE 8-1   **Embryonic Demise** *(continued)*

8-1C   Echogenic or "white" yolk sac associated with embryonic demise.

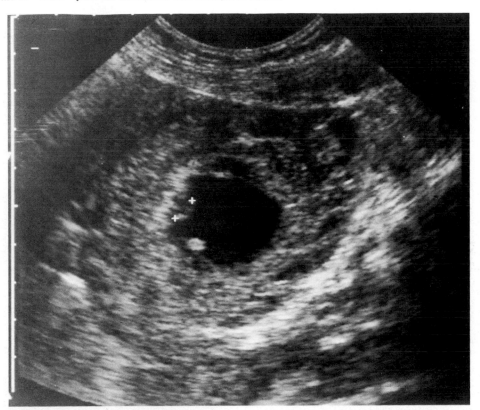

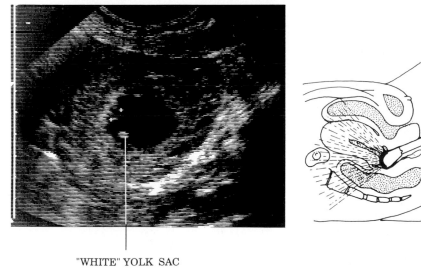

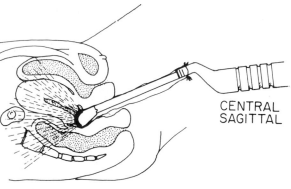

"WHITE" YOLK SAC

CENTRAL
SAGITTAL

(continued)

FIGURE 8-1   Embryonic Demise *(continued)*

8-1D   Relatively large gestational sac with deflated yolk sac in embryonic demise.

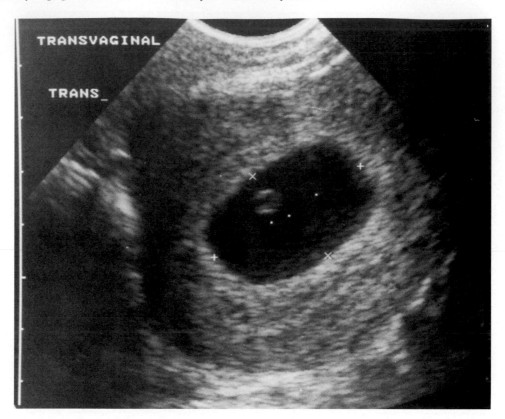

YOLK SAC

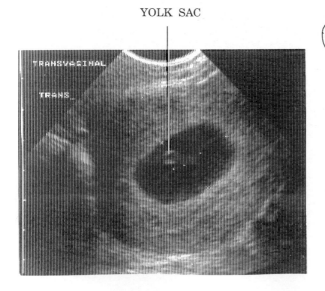

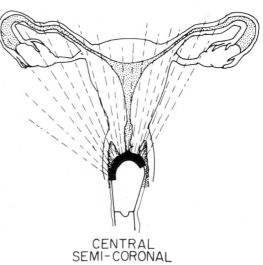

CENTRAL
SEMI-CORONAL

FIGURE 8-2 Abortion

8-2A Incomplete abortion appearing as echogenic tissue within the uterus.

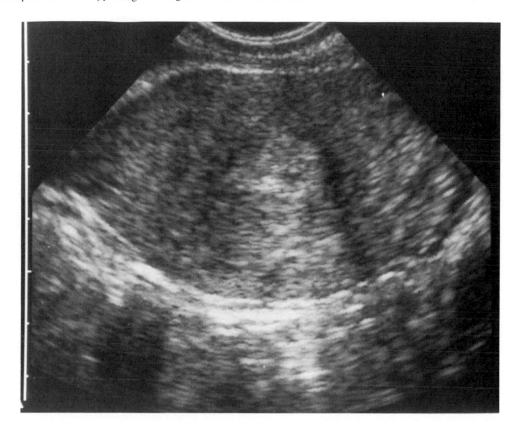

RETAINED CHORIODECIDUA

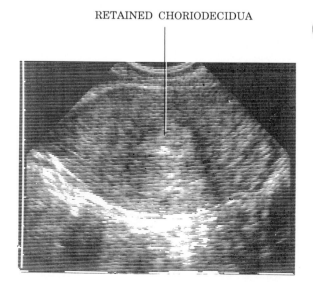
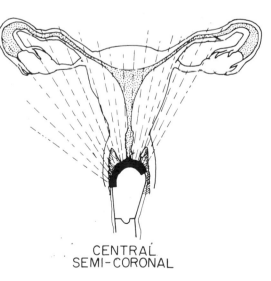

CENTRAL
SEMI-CORONAL

(continued)

FIGURE 8-2   Abortion (*continued*)

8-2B   Incomplete abortion with choriodecidua with lower uterine lumen.

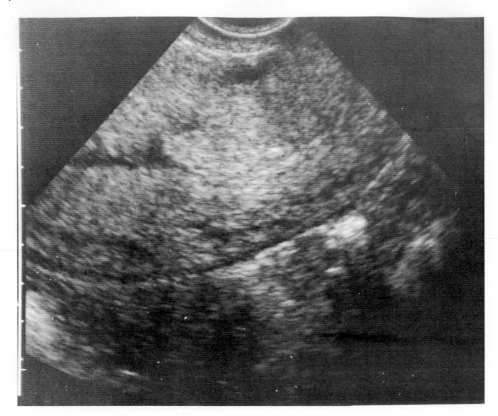

RETAINED CHORIODECIDUA

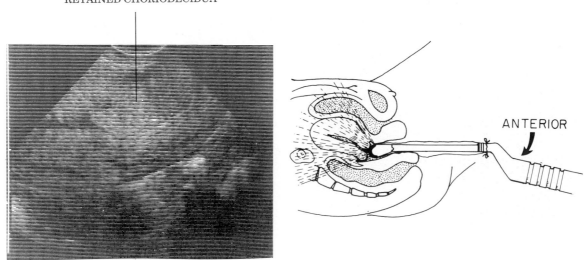

FIGURE 8-2   Abortion *(continued)*

8-2C   Abortion-in-progress showing choriodecidua within lower uterine lumen.

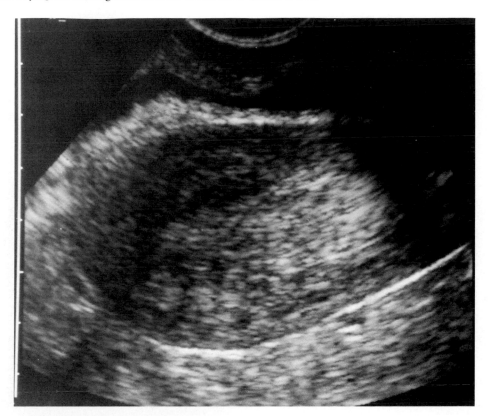

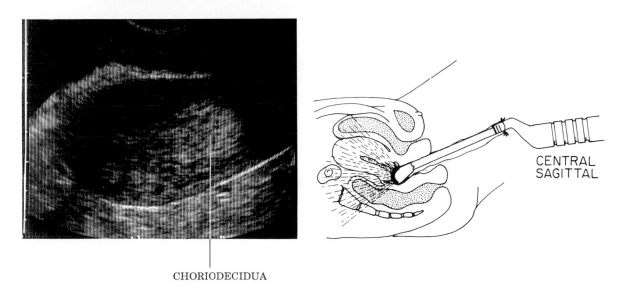

CHORIODECIDUA

CENTRAL
SAGITTAL

(continued)

FIGURE 8-2   Abortion *(continued)*

8-2D   Completed abortion showing closely opposed, thin endometrial interfaces.

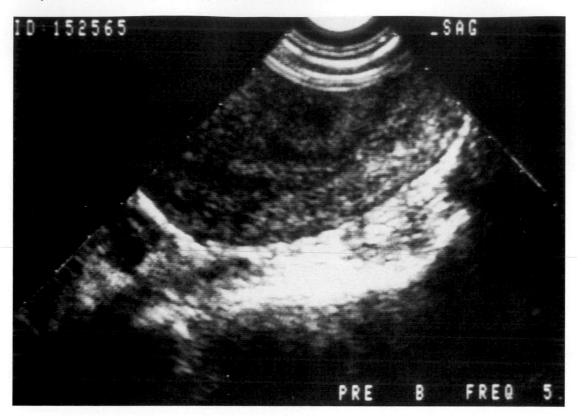

ENDOMETRIUM

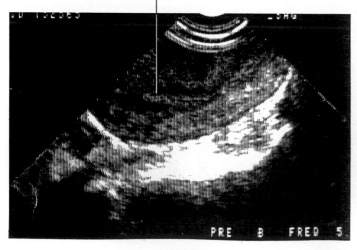

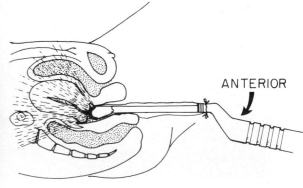

ANTERIOR

FIGURE 8-2   Abortion *(continued)*

8-2E   Blighted twin in empty sac adjacent to living embryo within intact gestational sac.

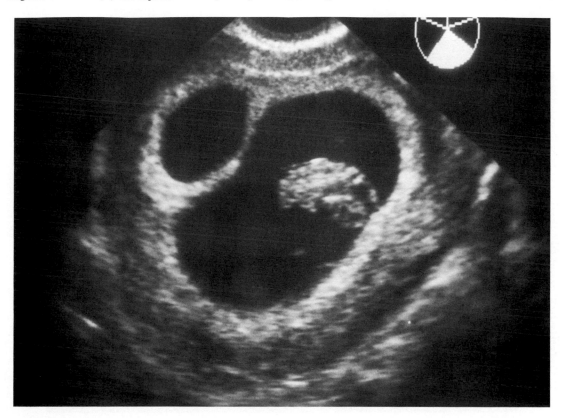

BLIGHTED TWIN

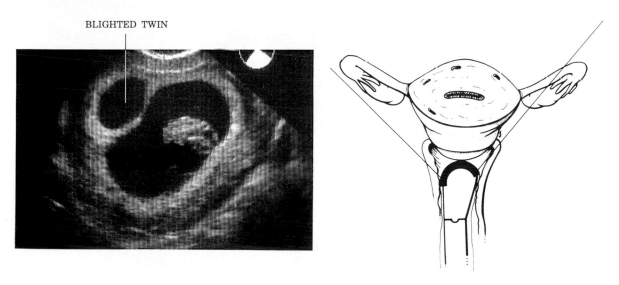

(continued)

FIGURE 8-2   Abortion *(continued)*

8-2F   Hydropic yolk sac associated with embryonic demise.

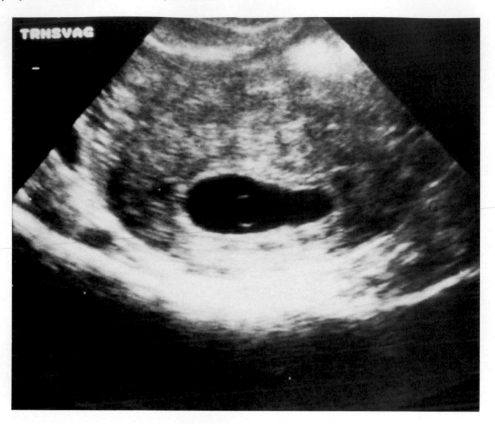

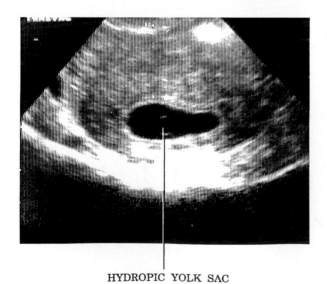

HYDROPIC YOLK SAC

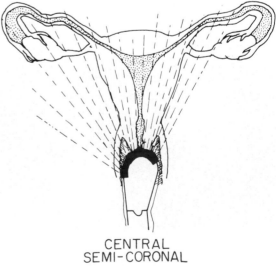

CENTRAL
SEMI-CORONAL

FIGURE 8-3   Other Conditions Associated with Bleeding

8-3A   Early molar pregnancy (gestational trophoblastic disease) simulating the appearance of an incomplete abortion.

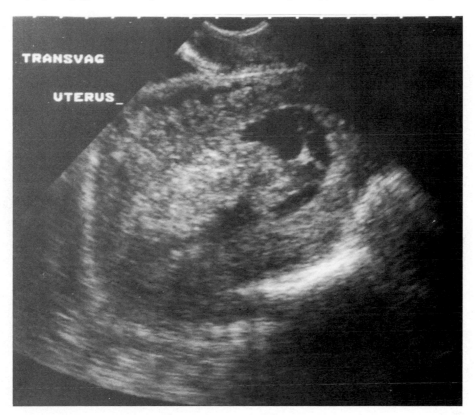

MOLAR TISSUE

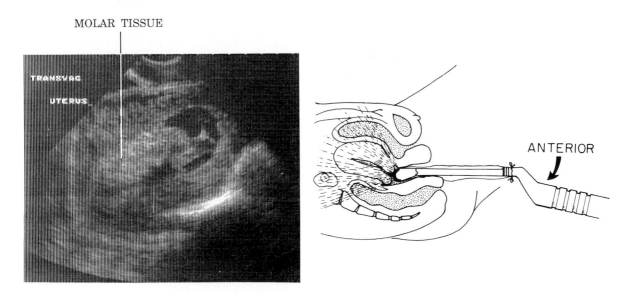

ANTERIOR

(continued)

FIGURE 8-3   Other Conditions Associated with Bleeding *(continued)*

8-3B   Retrochorionic hemorrhage surrounding a gestational sac containing a living embryo.

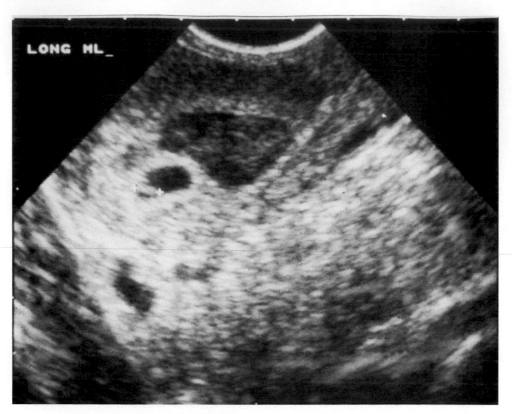

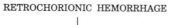

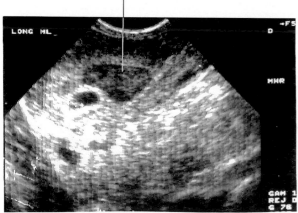

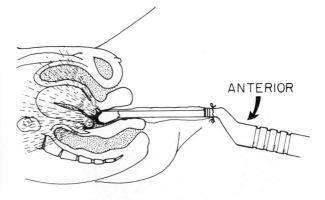

FIGURE 8-4   Ectopic Pregnancy—Uterine Findings

8-4A   Decidual thickening.

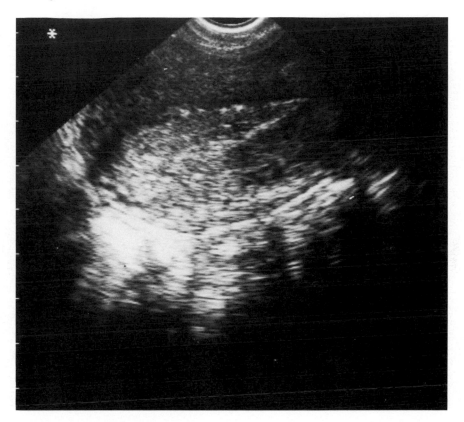

DECIDUALIZED ENDOMETRIUM

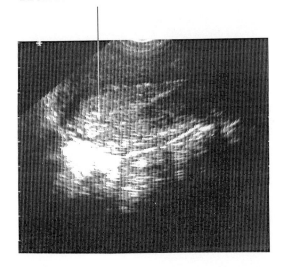

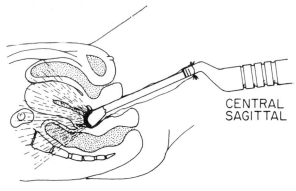

CENTRAL SAGITTAL

(continued)

FIGURE 8-4 Ectopic Pregnancy—Uterine Findings *(continued)*

8-4B Necrotic decidua with several hypoechoic areas (courtesy of R. Pennell, MD).

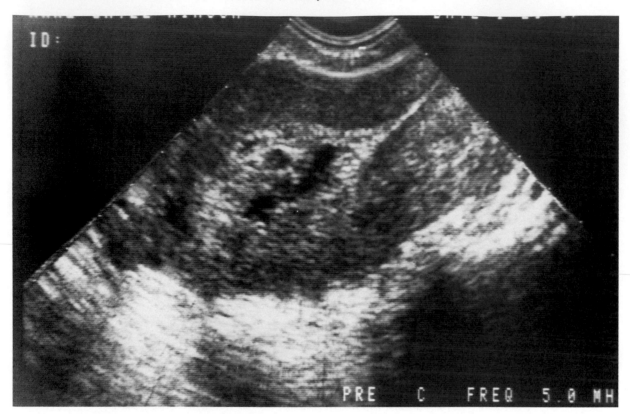

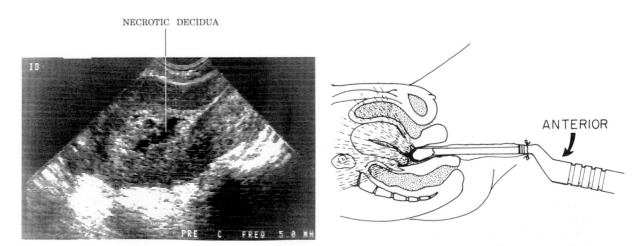

NECROTIC DECIDUA

ANTERIOR

FIGURE 8-4   Ectopic Pregnancy—Uterine Findings *(continued)*

8-4C   Pseudosac showing irregular decidual thickening. In addition, there is fluid in the cul-de-sac.

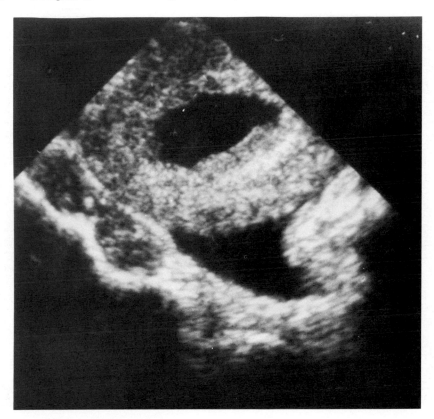

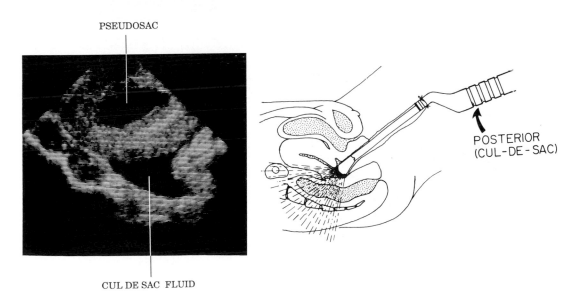

PSEUDOSAC

CUL DE SAC FLUID

POSTERIOR
(CUL-DE-SAC)

(continued)

FIGURE 8-4   Ectopic Pregnancy—Uterine Findings *(continued)*

8-4D   Pseudosac resulting from fluid accumulation within the uterine lumen.

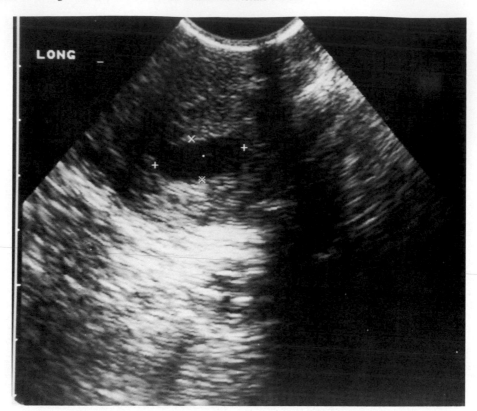

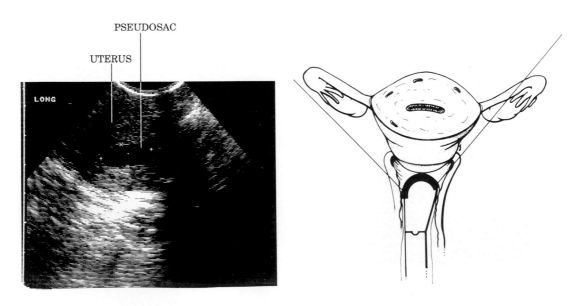

FIGURE 8-4   Ectopic Pregnancy—Uterine Findings *(continued)*

8-4E   Pseudosac with concentric and thin decidual thickening.

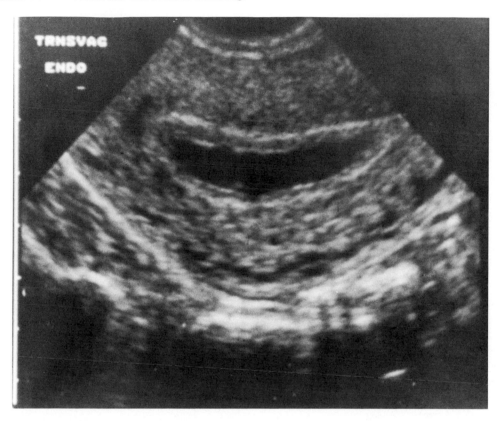

UTERUS

PSEUDOSAC

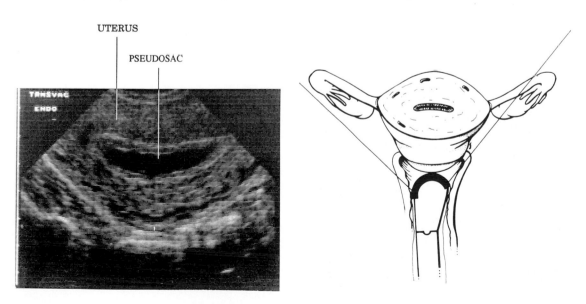

(continued)

FIGURE 8-4   Ectopic Pregnancy—Uterine Findings *(continued)*

8-4F   Hemorrhage within pseudosac of advanced ectopic pregnancy.

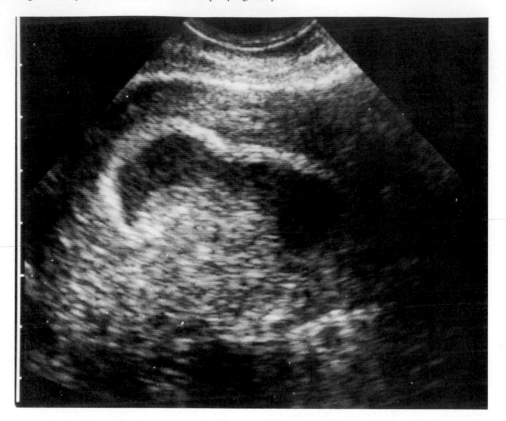

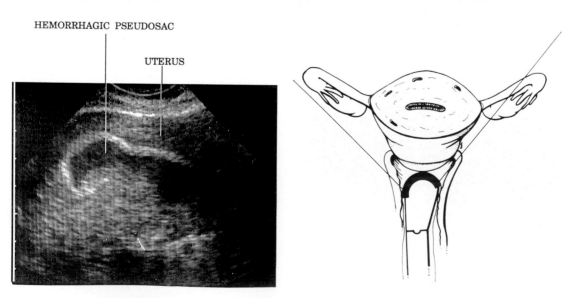

FIGURE 8-5   Ectopic Pregnancy—Adnexal Findings

8-5A "Tubal ring" representing an unruptured ectopic pregnancy in the left uterine tube. Laparoscopic appearance of unruptured ectopic pregnancy as a bulge in the left fallopian tube (arrow) (courtesy of C. Herbert, MD).

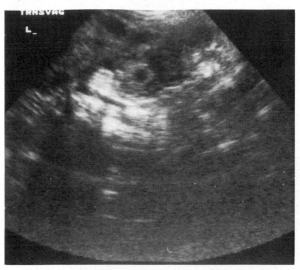
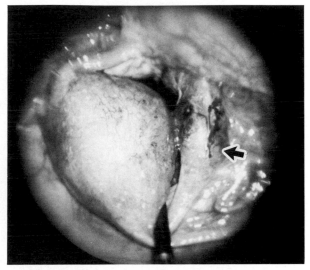

UNRUPTURED ECTOPIC

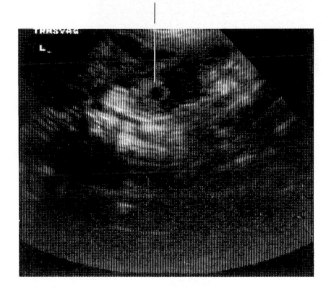
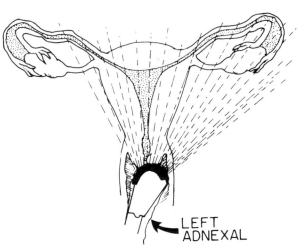

LEFT ADNEXAL

(continued)

FIGURE 8-5   **Ectopic Pregnancy—Adnexal Findings** *(continued)*

8-5B   Unruptured ectopic pregnancy adjacent to the nongravid uterus.

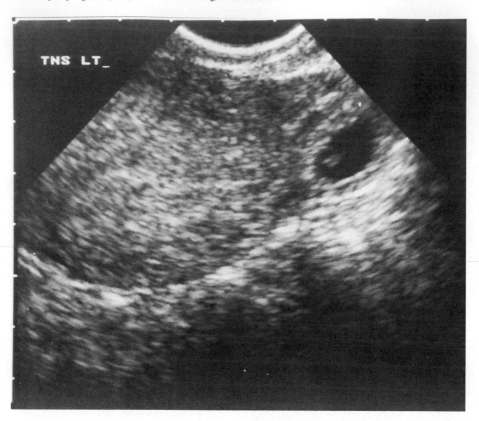

UTERUS

UNRUPTURED ECTOPIC

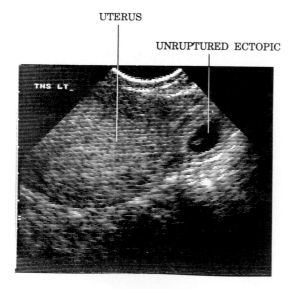

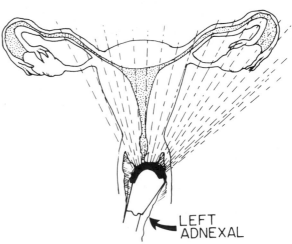

LEFT ADNEXAL

FIGURE 8-5   Ectopic Pregnancy—Adnexal Findings *(continued)*

8-5C   Unruptured ectopic pregnancy (seen in Fig. 8-5*B*) containing embryo with heart motion as shown on M-mode.

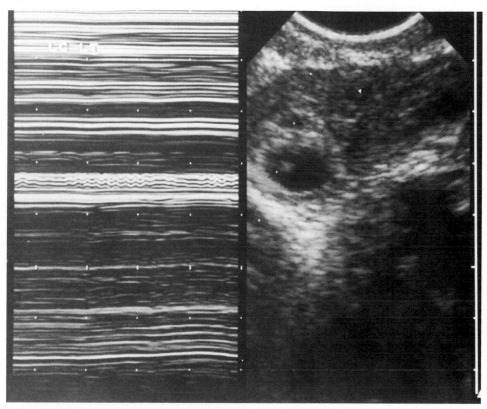

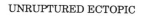
UNRUPTURED ECTOPIC

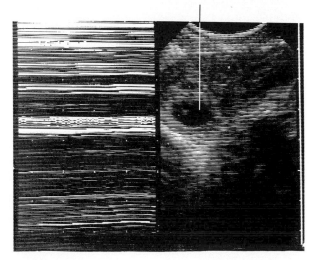

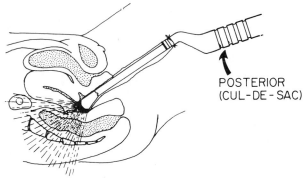
POSTERIOR
(CUL-DE-SAC)

(continued)

FIGURE 8-5   **Ectopic Pregnancy—Adnexal Findings** *(continued)*

8-5D   Unruptured ectopic pregnancy surrounded by thickened tubal wall.

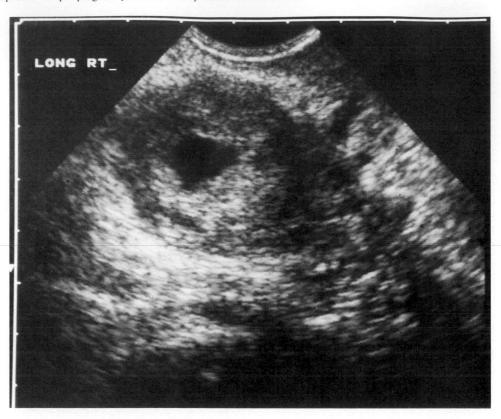

UNRUPTURED ECTOPIC

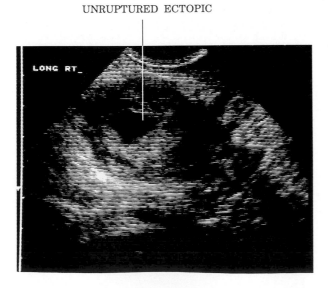

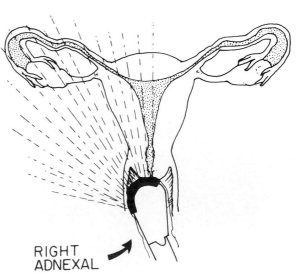

RIGHT
ADNEXAL

FIGURE 8-5   Ectopic Pregnancy—Adnexal Findings *(continued)*

8-5E   Unruptured ectopic pregnancy appearing as tubal mass. Cul-de-sac fluid resulted from blood oozing from the fimbriated end of the tube.

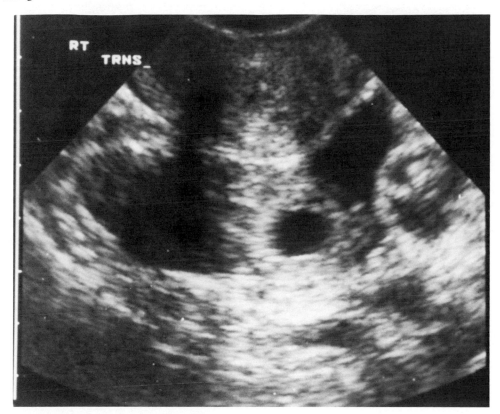

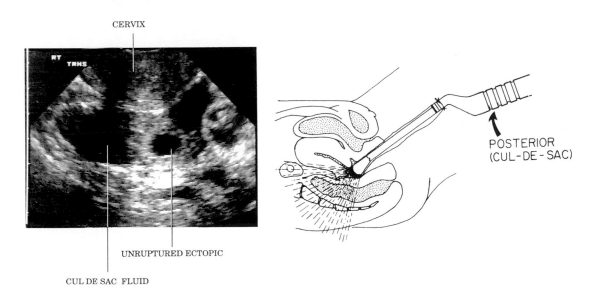

CERVIX

UNRUPTURED ECTOPIC

CUL DE SAC FLUID

POSTERIOR
(CUL-DE-SAC)

(continued)

FIGURE 8-5   Ectopic Pregnancy—Adnexal Findings *(continued)*

8-5F   Ruptured ectopic pregnancy resulting in hematosalpinx.

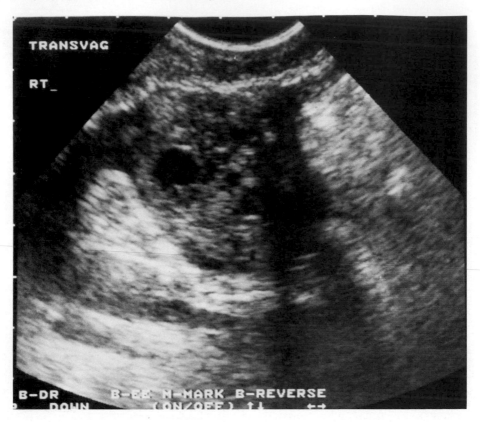

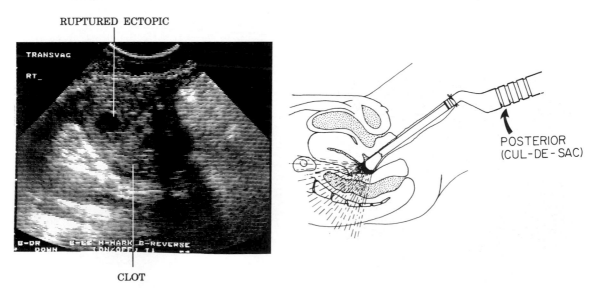

FIGURE 8-5   Ectopic Pregnancy—Adnexal Findings *(continued)*

8-5G   Corpus luteum adjacent to an unruptured ectopic pregnancy.

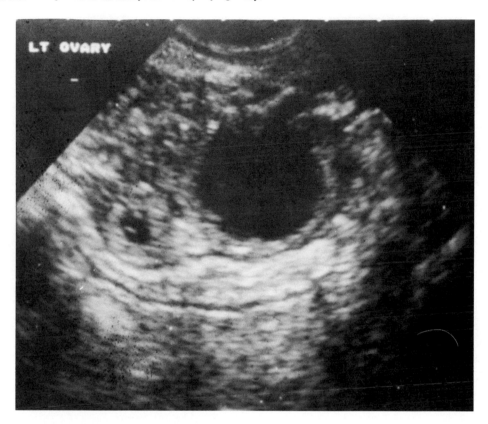

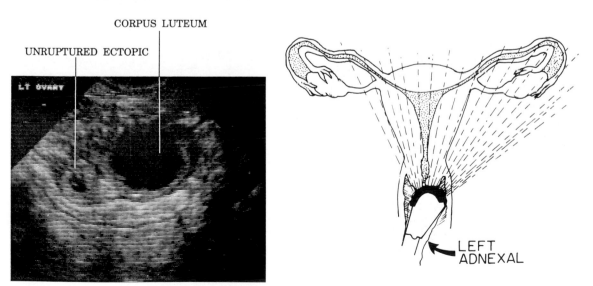

(continued)

FIGURE 8-5   Ectopic Pregnancy—Adnexal Findings *(continued)*

8-5H   Hemorrhagic corpus luteum with fine internal septae in a patient with an ectopic pregnancy.

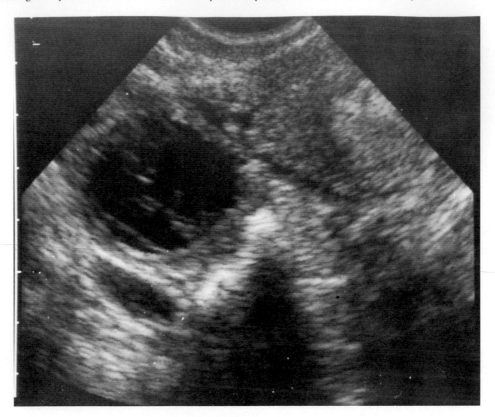

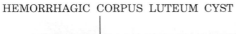
HEMORRHAGIC CORPUS LUTEUM CYST

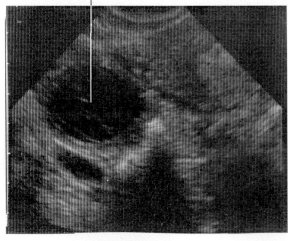

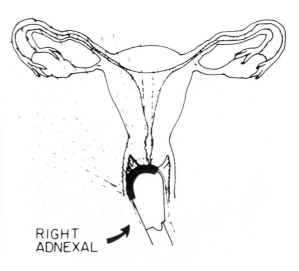
RIGHT
ADNEXAL

FIGURE 8-5   Ectopic Pregnancy—Adnexal Findings *(continued)*

8-51   Unruptured ectopic pregnancy with living 8-week-old fetus.

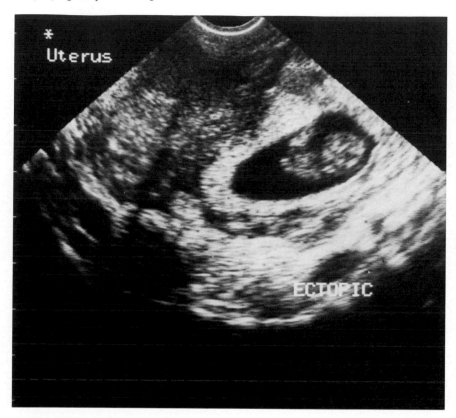

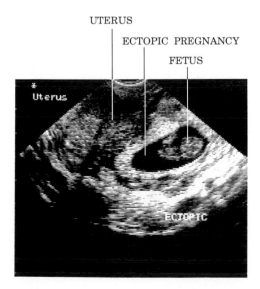

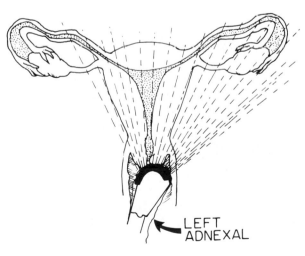

(continued)

FIGURE 8-5   Ectopic Pregnancy—Adnexal Findings *(continued)*

8-5J   Hematosalpinx and hematoperitoneum adjacent to corpus luteum cyst.

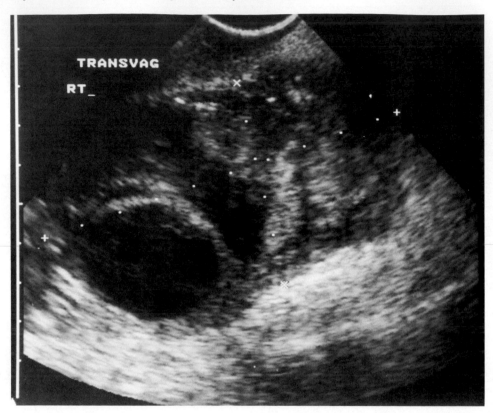

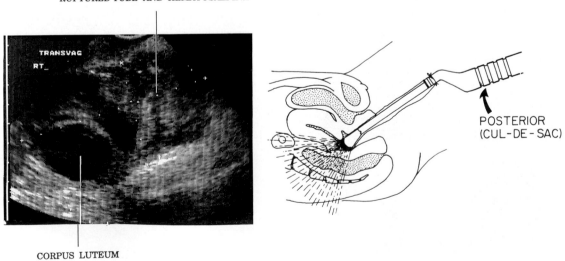

RUPTURED TUBE AND HEMATOSALPINX

CORPUS LUTEUM

POSTERIOR
(CUL-DE-SAC)

FIGURE 8-6   Cul-De-Sac Findings

8-6A   Echogenic or "particulate" intraperitoneal fluid surrounding unruptured ectopic pregnancy due to bleeding into the peritoneum from the tube. At laparoscopy, an unruptured ectopic pregnancy (arrow) was apparent within the intact left tube (courtesy of C. Herbert, MD).

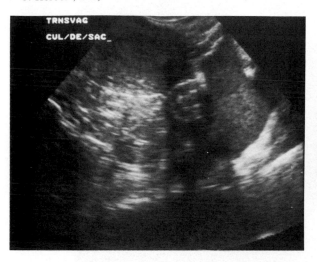

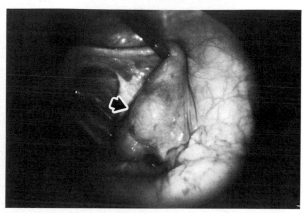

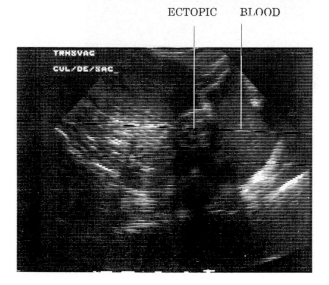

ECTOPIC   BLOOD

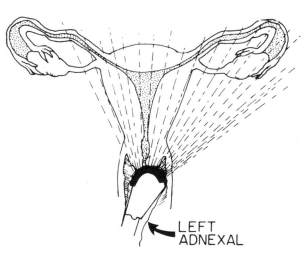

LEFT ADNEXAL

(continued)

FIGURE 8-6   Cul-De-Sac Findings *(continued)*

8-6B   Unruptured ectopic pregnancy within a hematosalpinx.

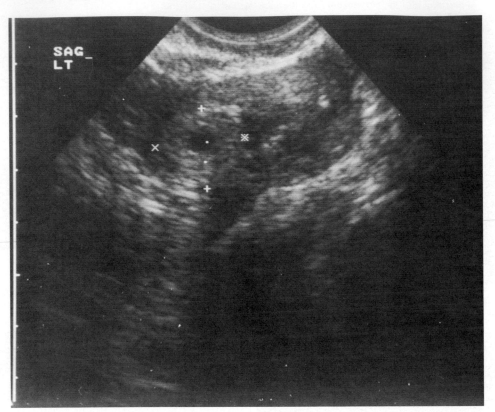

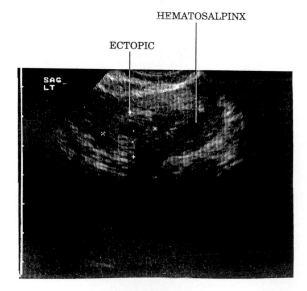

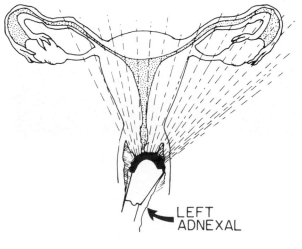

HEMATOSALPINX

ECTOPIC

LEFT ADNEXAL

FIGURE 8-7   Unusual Ectopic Pregnancies

8-7A   Cornual ectopic pregnancy eccentric to the endometrial lumen and within 5 mm of the uterine serosa.

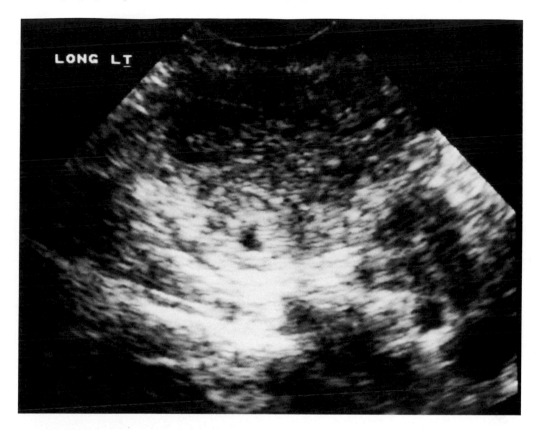

CORNUAL PREGNANCY

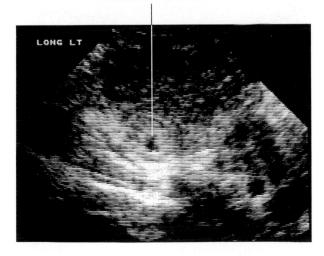

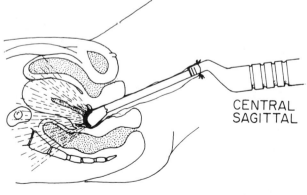

CENTRAL SAGITTAL

(continued)

FIGURE 8-7   Unusual Ectopic Pregnancies *(continued)*

8-7B   Cornual ectopic pregnancy with thick choriodecidual ring and lacunae.

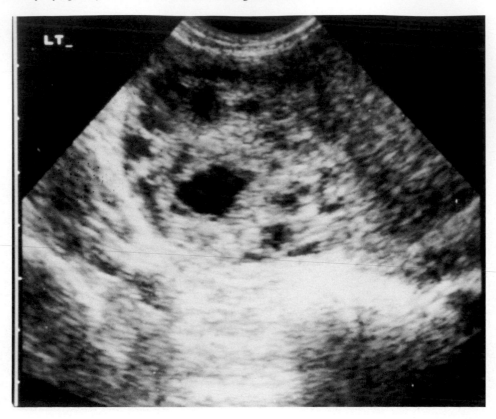

CORNUAL PREGNANCY

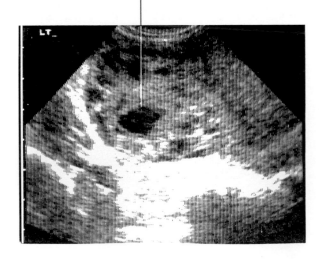

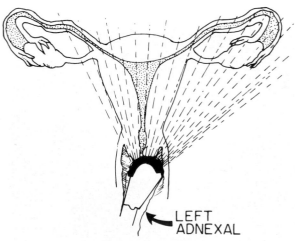

LEFT
ADNEXAL

FIGURE 8-7   Unusual Ectopic Pregnancies *(continued)*

8-7C   Cervical ectopic pregnancy in a patient with previous diethylstilbesterol (DES) exposure (also see Fig. 12-3 *A* to *D*).

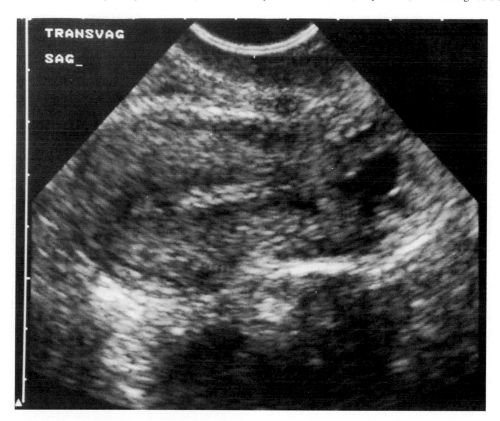

CERVICAL ECTOPIC

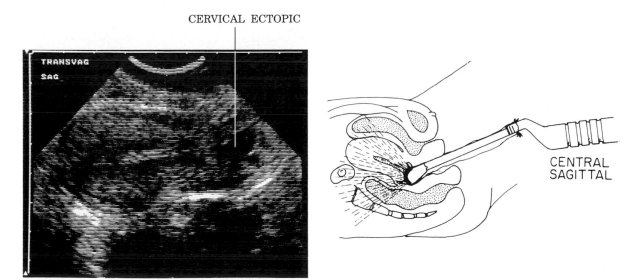

CENTRAL
SAGITTAL

(continued)

FIGURE 8-7   Unusual Ectopic Pregnancies *(continued)*

8-7D   Ovarian ectopic pregnancy with a dead embryo within gestational sac (courtesy of L. Needleman, MD).

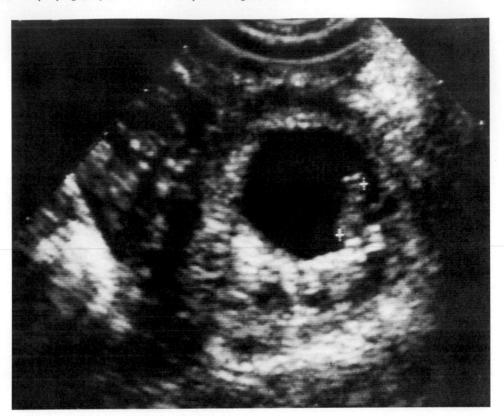

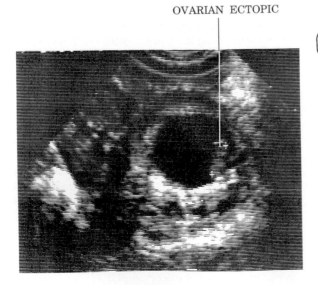

OVARIAN ECTOPIC

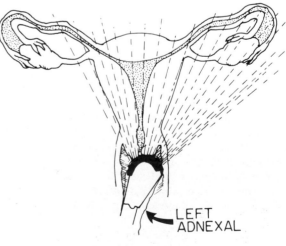

LEFT ADNEXAL

Chapter 9

The Lower Urinary Tract

M. J. Quinn, MRCOG

Introduction

Transvaginal sonography (TVS), using the appropriate equipment, is a simple, noninvasive technique for the assessment of the lower urinary tract in women with urinary incontinence (Quinn et al, 1988). High-frequency endoprobes with reduced external dimensions permit objective assessment of the bladder outlet at rest and during provocative maneuvers. Women without urinary symptoms have a well-supported bladder neck that remains closed during a cough. Opening of the bladder neck with concurrent urinary leakage during a cough, establishes a diagnosis of "genuine" stress incontinence (GSI) (Quinn et al, 1989).

Symptoms and signs may not establish the underlying cause of lower urinary tract symptoms and urodynamic investigations have been developed as an objective method of determining their cause (Enhorning, 1961; Bates et al, 1970; Hilton and Stanton, 1981). Twin-channel subtraction cystometry defines detrusor instability (DI) whereas synchronous videocystourethrography (VCUG) remains the standard for the diagnosis of genuine stress incontinence (Versi and Cardozo, 1986). These investigations are invasive and require established facilities and experienced staff to perform and interpret them (Stanton, 1983). Limited sensitivity and specificity of some aspects of urodynamic testing have been demonstrated (Richardson, 1986) and their reproducibility has not been established since most women are unwilling to undergo repetitive testing. For these reasons, they have not been universally accepted and there is divergence of opinion as to which patients may benefit (Shah, 1984; Jarvis et al, 1980; Benness, 1989; Stanton et al, 1988).

Previous radiologic techniques, notably bead-chain cystourethrography (BCUG), provide indirect images of the anatomic relationships although dynamic assessment is limited to the displacement of the bladder neck during provocative maneuvers (Green, 1962). Specific anatomic configurations have not proven to be specific for a diagnosis of GSI although it is clear that some typical patterns exist (Hodgkinson, 1970). Videocystourethrography includes imaging of the bladder neck and synchronous pressure measurements but requires urethral catheterization and radiologic facilities (Bates et al, 1970). Ultrasound has been proposed as a suitable alternative technique and abdominal, perineal, and rectal routes have been investigated (Brown et al, 1985; Gordon et al, 1989; Richmond et al, 1986). Lack of image resolution, distortion of the anatomic field, and limited patient acceptance have restricted their development. The vaginal route ensures the endoprobe is adjacent to the important landmarks without discomfort to the patient (Quinn et al, 1988). An offset field, high operating frequency, and reduced external dimensions ensure enhanced resolution of the image without distortion of the anatomic features. In contrast to BCUG, the effect of an increase in intraabdominal pressure on the continence mechanism and the presence or absence of urinary leakage are directly visible. Each scan may be completed in 5 minutes without urethral catheterization, contrast medium, and radiologic facilities (Quinn et al, 1988).

The primary requirement of a new technique is to differentiate GSI from DI since they represent the most common urinary complaints and their treatment differs markedly (Hilton, 1987). In many patients the two conditions coexist, and it has been argued that the determination of the presence or absence of GSI should be the central issue, since in most cases an accurate suprapubic operation cures both conditions (McGuire and Savastano, 1985). Comparison of the anatomic consequences of different suprapubic operations is an additional benefit of the technique since the position of the bladder neck relative to the inferior border of the symphysis pubis may be objectively assessed (Quinn et al, 1989). Despite the improved success rates of suprapubic surgery, a proportion of patients have persistent or recurrent postoperative symptoms, the cause of which has not been elucidated (Hertogs and Stanton, 1985). Controlled studies determine the precise role of trans-

FIGURE 9-1 The operating characteristics of the endoprobe are critical for imaging the lower urinary tract. The endoprobe has an operating frequency of 7 Mhz and scans through an arc of 112 degrees over a focal range of 1 to 6 cm. The field is offset and the crystal has a frame rate of 20 frames per second so that the dynamic effects of a cough on the continence mechanism may be visualized.

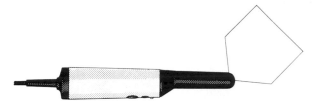

vaginal ultrasound in the management of patients with lower urinary tract symptoms.

Technique

Successful imaging of the lower urinary tract requires equipment capable of static and dynamic assessment in both recumbent and sitting positions. A 7 MHz me-

chanical sector scanner with an offset field (45 degrees), wide field angle (112 degrees), high frame rate (20 Hz), and reduced, external dimensions (maximum diameter 22 mm) is important (Bruel & Kjaer 8537; Fig. 9-1). These specifications ensure a sagittal section of the anterior pelvis in the plane of the symphysis pubis. The high frame rate ensures imaging of the continence mechanism during a cough, and the reduced external dimensions avoid any distortion of the anatomic features. Linear array systems may provide appropriate images of the lower urinary tract although they are most often available at frequencies of 5 MHz with a convex array and corresponding external shape that prevent satisfactory resolution of the anatomic features.

Full assessment includes history, examination, and ultrasound scanning in both recumbent and sitting positions with a full bladder. After explanation of the procedure, the patient assumes a recumbent position on a flat couch. The endoprobe is placed in the finger of a sterile disposable glove and liberally covered with coupling gel. The first structures to be visualized are the symphysis pubis and the pubic ramus with the bladder and urethra immediately posterior to the symphysis (Figs. 9-2, 9-3). Examination in the recumbent position permits accurate assessment of the relative

FIGURE 9-2 The bladder appears as a hypoechoic structure because of the stored urine. The course of the urethra is indicated by the acoustic characteristics of the adjacent tissues. In the midline sagittal plane the symphysis pubis appears as a dense, uniform, hyperechoic feature. In all scans the longitudinal axis of the patient extends from the top, left corner of the scan (head) to the bottom right corner (feet). B, bladder; BN, bladder neck; SP, symphysis pubis.

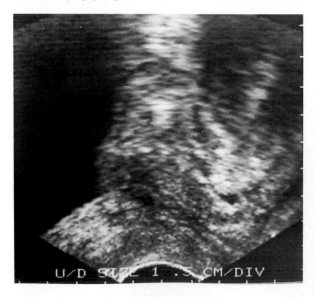
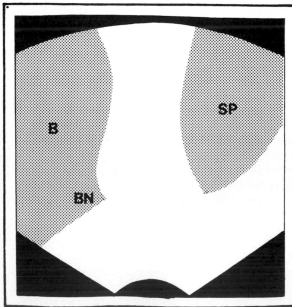

FIGURE 9-3 The same patient as in Figure 9-2 is shown with the bladder emptied and the pubic bone scanned in an oblique plane. The trabecular bone of the body of the pubis appears as a hypoechoic feature in contrast to the hyperechoic, cortical bone of the inferior border. BN, bladder neck; PR, pubic ramus.

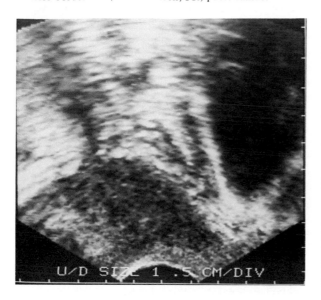 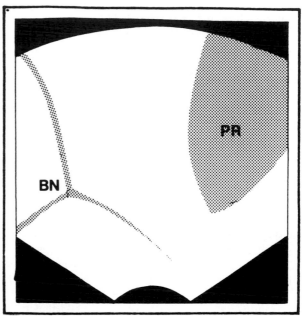

positions of the bladder neck and the inferior border of the symphysis pubis in the sagittal plane. Examination in the sitting position during provocative maneuvers is a sensitive technique for the diagnosis of GSI (Quinn et al, 1989). The patient is invited to sit on a commode with a sheet over the lower half of her body; she places the endoprobe at the introitus, where it is held in the correct plane by the examiner so that the patient may sit erect to carry out a series of provocative maneuvers. Opening of the bladder neck with urinary leakage concurrent with a cough establishes a diagnosis of GSI (Quinn et al, 1987).

Limiting features of the technique include inadequate bladder filling, moderate or severe prolapse of the anterior vaginal wall, and distortion of the anatomic features. Minor degrees of prolapse do not restrict ultrasound scanning although moderate or severe prolapse prevents examination with the patient in the sitting position. The precise effect of the endoprobe on adjacent tissues is visible throughout the scan and may be observed on the ultrasound monitor. Reorientation of the endoprobe avoids any distorting effect. Patient acceptance is enhanced by the reduced external dimensions and the offset field that ensures the tip of the endoprobe is placed no more than 1 to 2 cm within the vagina throughout the examination.

Sonographic Anatomy of the Lower Urinary Tract

Sonographic appearances of the lower urinary tract depend on the differing acoustic impedances of the different structures—urine, cartilage, trabecular and cortical bone. Additional information may be gained by introducing foreign materials with an independent acoustic pattern, such as catheters or microtransducers.

SYMPHYSIS PUBIS AND PUBIC RAMUS

The symphysis pubis is a secondary cartilaginous joint with sonographic appearances determined by the pad of cartilage connecting the pubic bones. Cartilage appears as a dense, homogeneous, echogenic pattern differentiated from the surrounding connective tissue by the shape of the inferior half of the pubis and its immobility during a cough or Valsalva maneuver (see Fig. 9-2). The symphysis is a uniform midline structure that provides a fixed reference point from which reproducible measurements may be made. The pubis adjacent to the symphysis is composed of trabecular bone with a dense inferior cortex that appears as a hypoechoic body with a hyperechoic inferior border (see Fig. 9-3).

THE BLADDER AND URETHRA

The position of the bladder is identified by the hypo-echoic appearance of the stored urine (see Fig. 9-2). The course of the urethra is identified by the acoustic properties of the adjacent tissues including its vascular supply (see Figs. 9-2, 9-3). The bladder neck may refer to a number of different structures. Radiologically it is the junction of the bladder and the urethra; histologically it is the junction of squamous and transitional epithelium; urodynamically it denotes a gradient in pressure. For the purposes of this chapter it represents the junction of the urethra and a comfortably full bladder (200 to 400 mL).

Sonographic Appearances of Urinary Incontinence

In patients without urinary symptoms dynamic assessment of the bladder neck in the sitting position may be associated with slight posterior or inferior displacement of the bladder neck, but there is no associated leakage of urine (Quinn et al, 1988; Quinn et al, 1989).

Examination in the sitting position establishes the presence or absence of genuine stress incontinence (Quinn et al, 1989). Opening of the bladder neck and proximal urethra, with urinary leakage concurrent with a cough, is the hallmark of GSI (Fig. 9-4). This finding is sensitive and specific for the diagnosis of GSI, differentiating this condition from detrusor instability in a consecutive series of 124 patients (Quinn et al, 1989). Patients with relatively minor symptoms of stress incontinence, for example, urinary leakage during vigorous exercise, may not demonstrate these sonographic findings since the increase in intraabdominal pressure cannot be reproduced in the testing situation. Downward displacement of the bladder neck is observed although this is not specific to establish a diagnosis of GSI (Hodgkinson, 1970).

Opening of the bladder neck resulting from detrusor instability occurs under different circumstances and in a different fashion from that associated with GSI (Fig. 9-5). Detrusor instability may be provoked by a change in position, hand-washing, coughing, or bladder filling. Much of the justification or objective assessment of patients with urinary incontinence derives from the observation that a cough may provoke urinary leakage in patients with detrusor instability and this may be mistaken for GSI. Cough-induced instability is differentiated from urinary leakage resulting from GSI since there is a clear interval between the increase in intraabdominal pressure and subsequent opening of the bladder neck that may be recognized during ultrasound examination.

FIGURE 9-5 Opening of the bladder neck and urinary leakage associated with detrusor instability is different in timing and appearance to that of stress incontinence.

FIGURE 9-4 Genuine stress incontinence. Opening of the bladder neck and proximal urethra with urinary leakage concurrent with a cough.

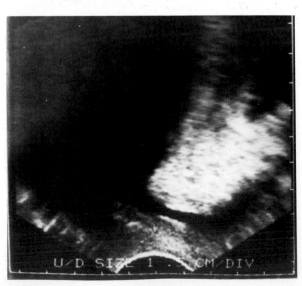

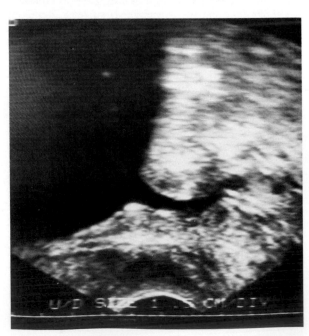

The Anatomic Effects of Suprapubic Operations

Many operations have been devised for the treatment of urinary stress incontinence. With the recognition that the abdominal operations have more consistent results than vaginal procedures (Stanton and Cardozo, 1979), different forms of suprapubic operations have become increasingly popular. The refinement of the surgical repertoire has established three main categories of suprapubic operation: retropubic urethropexy, in the form of colposuspension (Burch, 1961) or Marshall-Marchetti-Krantz procedure (Krantz, 1980); needle suspension procedures (Pereyra, 1959; Raz, 1981; Stamey, 1980); and sling operations (Hohenfellner and Petri, 1980) All these operations elevate the bladder neck and provide support in its new position so as to restore continence. Despite improved results a proportion of patients have persistent or recurrent urinary symptoms after these procedures.

After colposuspension different anatomic configurations are associated with successful and unsuccessful results. Successful outcomes are associated with elevation and support of the bladder neck so that an increase in intraabdominal pressure does not cause displacement or opening of the bladder neck (Fig. 9-6). Unsuccessful outcomes, including early and late recurrent stress incontinence, frequency–urgency syndrome, and persistent urinary incontinence, are associated with four different anatomic configurations. Recurrent stress incontinence (RSI) occurs in two situations. Early RSI occurs in the immediate postoperative period and results from primary failure of the supporting sutures. Any increase in intraabdominal pressure leads to downward displacement and opening of the bladder neck with a cough. Late RSI in the early postmenopausal years may occur after an apparently successful operation some years before menopause. Examination of the patient shows that although the sutures are intact there is sufficient loss of support to allow urinary leakage with a cough. Inaccurate placement of the supporting sutures relative to the bladder neck may be associated with either persistent incontinence or persistent postoperative frequency and urgency (Figs. 9-7, 9-8). If the sutures are placed adjacent to the vaginal vault, securing them to the iliopectineal ligament causes indentation of the bladder base by the vaginal shelf (see Fig. 9-7), there is no elevation of the bladder neck, and stress incontinence persists. Placing the sutures between the vaginal vault and the bladder neck leads to indentation of trigone by the vaginal shelf (see Fig. 9-8), persistent symptoms of frequency and urgency, and de novo appearance of detrusor instability (Jarvis, 1981; Langer et al, 1988). This observation calls into question the frequently cited

FIGURE 9-6 Successful colposuspension. The bladder neck has been elevated to a new position behind the symphysis pubis. Nonabsorbable suture material in the vaginal fornices and the iliopectineal ligament appears as a hyperechoic feature. The symphysis pubis, bladder floor, neck, and urethra are outlined.

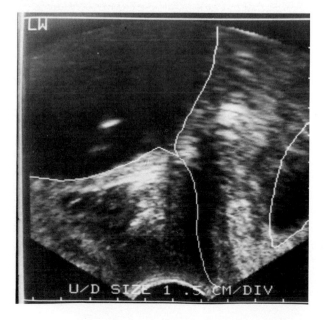

FIGURE 9-7 Persistent stress incontinence after colposuspension. The supporting sutures have been placed closer to the vaginal vault than the bladder neck, with the result that there has been no elevation of the bladder neck and the vaginal shelf indents the bladder base.

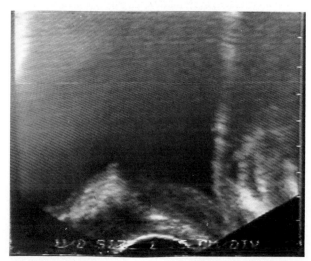

FIGURE 9-8 Frequency–urgency syndrome after colposuspension. The vaginal shelf is beneath the trigone rather than at the level of the bladder neck.

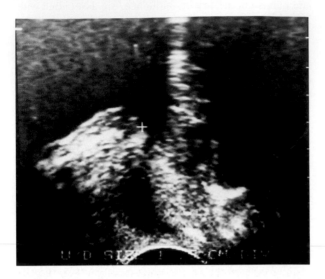

FIGURE 9-9 Successul Stamey needle-suspension. The bladder neck is elevated above the inferior border of the symphysis pubis.

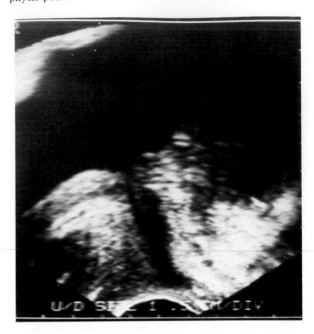

statement that suprapubic surgery worsens detrusor instability, since it is clear that a well-executed suprapubic operation cures most patients with combined symptoms of stress incontinence and detrusor instability. Inaccurate placement of the supporting sutures raises a vaginal shelf beneath the trigone that is consistently associated with the postoperative development of detrusor instability (Quinn et al, 1989; Jarvis, 1981; Langer et al, 1988).

Successful outcomes after needle-suspension operations are associated with anatomic appearances similar to those of colposuspension where the bladder neck is elevated and there is no downward displacement with a cough or Valsalva maneuver (Figs. 9-9, 9-10). They have been associated with a significant incidence of early recurrent stress incontinence in the immediate postoperative period. This results from ipsilateral or bilateral failure of the supporting sutures and recurrent stress incontinence.

Summary

TVS is a simple, noninvasive technique for the objective assessment of the lower urinary tract in patients with urinary incontinence. In contrast to preceding radiologic techniques, TVS produces direct dynamic images of the effects of provocative maneuvers on the continence mechanism without urethral catheterization and exposure to x-rays. Equipment specifications are important in providing high-resolution images without distortion of the anatomic features, and these include an operating

FIGURE 9-10 The same patient as Fig. 9-9 during a Valsalva maneuver. The bladder neck remains in a fixed position although the bladder base rotates towards the symphysis.

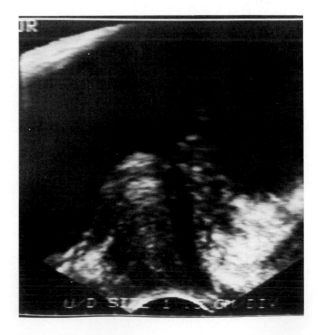

FIGURE 9-11   TVS of Urethra with Probe Placed at the Introitus

9-11A   Prior to Q-tip insertion, the urethra is closed and at proper angle relative to symphysis pubis.

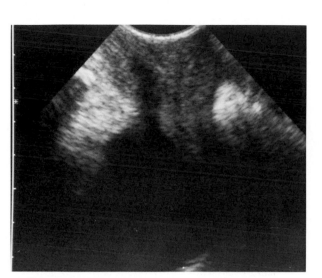
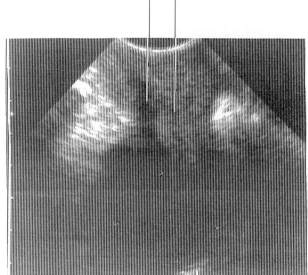

SYMPHYSIS PUBIS   URETHRA

9-11B   After Q-tip inserted within urethra showing angle of the urethra to the symphysis pubis.

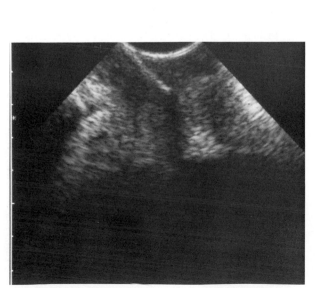
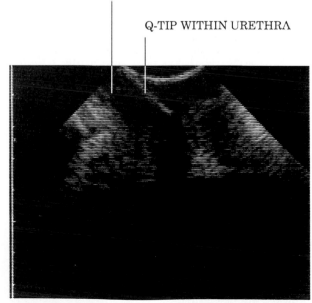

SYMPHYSIS PUBIS

Q-TIP WITHIN URETHRA

frequency of 7 MHz, an offset field, reduced external dimensions, and a high frame rate. Examination in the sitting position is a sensitive and specific technique for the diagnosis of genuine stress incontinence. Examination in the recumbent position permits accurate determination of the position of the bladder neck relative to the inferior border of the symphysis pubis. Persistent or recurrent postoperative symptoms after suprapubic surgery are associated with a variety of anatomic configurations caused by inaccurate surgical technique. Preexisting detrusor instability combined with stress incontinence may be cured by an accurate suprapubic operation, whereas an inaccurate operation may cause postoperative detrusor instability.

In its present format, TVS will not replace all aspects of traditional urodynamic studies although it should avoid many time-consuming and invasive investigations in patients who have urinary incontinence.

References

Bates CP, Whiteside CG, Turner-Warwick R. Synchronous cine/pressure/flow cystourethrography with special reference to stress and urge incontinence. *Br J Urol* 1970; 42:714–723.

Benness CJ, Barnick CG, Cardozo L. Is there a place for routine videocystourethrography in the assessment of lower urinary tract dysfunction? *Neurourol Urodyn* 1989; 8:291–297.

Brown MC, Sutherst JR, Murray A, Richmond DH. Potential use of ultrasound in place of x-ray fluoroscopy in urodynamics. *Br J. Urol* 1985;57:88–90.

Burch JC. Urethrovaginal fixation to Cooper's ligament for correction of stress incontinence, cystocoele and prolapse. *Am J Obstet Gynecol* 1961;117:805–813.

Enhorning G. Simultaneous recording of intravesical and intraurethral pressure. *Acta Chir Scand* 1961;125(suppl):276.

Gordon D, Pearce M, Norton P, Stanton SL. Comparison of ultrasound and lateral chain urethrocystography in the determination of bladder neck descent. *Am J Obstet Gynecol* 1989;160:182–186.

Green T. Development of a plan for the diagnosis and treatment of urinary stress incontinence. *Am J Obstet Gynecol* 1962; 83:632–648.

Hertogs K, Stanton SL. Lateral bead-chain urethrocystography after successful and unsuccessful colposuspension. *Br J Obstet Gynaecol* 1985;92:1179–1185.

Hilton P, Stanton SL. Urethral pressure measurement by microtransducer. I. An analysis of variance; II. An analysis of rotation variations. In: Sundin T, Mattiasson A, eds. *Proceedings 11th Annual Meeting International Continence Society.* Lund, Sweden, 1981a:69.

Hilton P. Urinary incontinence in women. *Br Med J* 1987; 299:455–460.

Hodgkinson CP. Stress urinary incontinence–1970. *Am J Obstet Gynecol* 1970;108:1141–1168.

Hohenfellner R, Petri E. Sling procedures. In: Stanton SL, Tanagho E, eds. *Surgery of Female Incontinence.* New York: Springer-Verlag, 1980.

Jarvis GJ, Hall S, Stamp S, Millar DR, Johnson A. An assessment of urodynamic examination in incontinent women. *Br J Obstet Gynaecol* 1980;87:893–896.

Jarvis GJ. Detrusor muscle instability: a complication of surgery? *Am J Obstet Gynecol* 1981;139:219.

Krantz K. Marshall-Marchetti-Krantz procedure. In: Stanton SL, Tanagho E, eds. *Surgery of Female Incontinence.* Heidelberg: Springer, 1980:47–54.

Langer R, Ron-El R, Newman M, Herman A, Caspi E. Detrusor instability following colposuspension for urinary stress incontinence. *Br J Obstet Gynaecol* 1988;95:607–610.

McGuire EJ, Savastano JA. Stress incontinence and detrusor instability/urge incontinence. *Neurourol Urodynam* 1985; 4:313–316.

Nicholls DH. Vaginal prolapse affecting bladder function. *Clin Obstet Gynecol* 1985;12:449–464.

Pereyra AJ. A simplified surgical procedure for the correction of stress incontinence in women. *West J Surg* 1959;67:223.

Quinn MJ, Beynon J. Mortensen NM, Smith PJB. Transvaginal endosonography in the assessment of urinary stress incontinence. *Br J Urol* 1988;62:414–418.

Quinn MJ, Beynon J, Mortensen NM, Smith PJB. Vaginal endosonography in the postoperative assessment of colposuspension. *Br J Urol* 1989;63:295–300.

Quinn MJ, Farnsworth BA, Pollard WJ, Smith PJB, Stott MA. Vaginal ultrasound in the diagnosis of stress incontinence: a prospective comparison to urodynamic investigations. *Neuro Urodynam* 1989;8:291–297.

Raz S. Modified bladder neck suspension for female stress incontinence. *Urology* 1981;18:82.

Richardson DA. Value of the cough pressure profile in the evaluation of patients with stress incontinence. *Am J Obstet Gynecol* 1986;155:808–811.

Richmond DH, Sutherst JR, Brown MC. Screening of the bladder base and urethra using linear array transrectal ultrasound scanning. *J Clin Ultrasound* 1986;14:647–651.

Shah PJR. The assessment of patients with a view to urodynamics. In: Mundy A, Wein A, Stephenson T, eds. *Urodynamics: Principles, Practice and Application.* Edinburgh: Churchill-Livingston Pub; 1984;53–62.

Stamey T. Endoscopic suspension of the vesical neck. In: Stanton SL, Tanagho E, eds. *Surgery of Female Incontinence.* Heidelberg: Springer 1980:77–90.

Stanton SL, Cardozo L. Results of the colposuspension operation for incontinence and prolapse. *Br J Obstet Gynaecol* 1979;86:693–697.

Stanton SL. What is the place of urodynamic investigations in a district general hospital? *Br J Obstet Gynaecol* 1983; 90:97. Editorial.

Stanton SL, Krieger MS, Ziv E. Videocystourethrography: its role in the assessment of incontinence in the female. *Neurourol Urodynam* 1988;7:155–160.

Versi E, Cardozo L. Perineal pad weighing versus videographic analysis in genuine stress incontinence. *Br J Obstet Gynaecol* 1986;93:364–366.

Zacharin RF. The suspensory mechanism of the female urethra. *J Anat* 1963;97:423–427.

Chapter 10

The Cervix During Pregnancy

M. J. Quinn, MRCOG

Introduction

Abdominal ultrasound equipment, operating at frequencies of 3 to 5 MHz, requires the reduced acoustic impedance of a full bladder to image the cervix in a pregnant woman. The position of the uterus, interposed fetal anatomy, and distortion of the anatomic features by the distended, full bladder may prevent resolution of the anatomic features (Bernstine et al, 1981). Vaginal endoprobes, operating at 5 to 7 MHz, avoid the need for bladder filling and provide consistent images of the cervix, (Quinn et al, 1989). A 7-MHz mechanical sector scanner with an offset field (Bruel & Kjaer 8537) provides reproducible images without discomfort to the patient. Patient acceptance is enhanced by the smooth symmetrical shape and reduced external dimensions (maximum diameter 22 mm;—see Chapter 9).

Scanning Technique and Normal Anatomy

After a preliminary explanation of the technique, the patient is placed in the dorsal recumbent position, similar to that for digital vaginal examination. The endoprobe is placed in the finger of a sterile disposable glove and lubricated with coupling gel. With the bladder previously emptied, the endoprobe is placed within the introitus. The symphysis pubis, pubic ramus, urethra, and empty bladder are the first structures to be visualized. Advancing the endoprobe beyond the posterior limit of the empty bladder brings the lower uterine cavity into view. The cervix is identified by the many hypoechoic, mucus-producing follicles in its lateral border. Rotation of the endoprobe around its longitudinal axis identifies a single, sagittal plane in which the cervical canal may be imaged in its entirety (Fig. 10-1). The internal cervical os is identified at the proximal limit of the cervical canal against the hypoechoic background of the amniotic sac (Figs. 10-1, 10-2).

In early pregnancy the cervical canal is up to 5 cm in length and there is little difference between nulliparous and multiparous women (Quinn et al, 1989). As pregnancy advances, the lower segment forms and the internal cervical os becomes readily identifiable against the background of the amniotic sac. In the final weeks of pregnancy shortening and dilation occur, and the amniotic membranes and presenting fetal presenting part are distinguishable from the lower uterine segment (See Fig. 10-2). Low-lying placentae and their relationship to the internal cervical os may be distinguished from adjacent structures by their characteristic appearances (Fig. 10-3).

Although there are no established standards for abnormal cervical length throughout pregnancy, it is clear that cervical length of less than 2.5 to 3.0 cm and less than 1.5 cm in anteroposterior thickness should be followed closely for additional signs of actual dilation of the endocervical canal (Brown et al, 1986). Minimal dilation (less than 1 cm) of the endocervical canal can be observed in normal pregnancies after 34 to 36 weeks. The diagnosis of cervical incompetence should be based both on the dilation of the endocervical canal and shortening and thinning of the cervix.

Incompetent Cervix

Cervical incompetence is usually a clinical diagnosis suspected in women with a history of midtrimester loss. Preceding surgical operations in which the cervical canal is forcibly dilated have been implicated as causative factors although the effects of such damage have been difficult to detect with conventional techniques. Previous obstetric history is not a specific indicator of subsequent

FIGURE 10-1 The cervix in a pregnant woman imaged in the plane of the cervical canal has a homogeneous, echogenic appearance in contrast to a plane adjacent to the midline, where large numbers of hypoechoic, mucus-producing follicles are visible. The cervical canal is a hypoechoic feature extending from the internal (large arrow) to the external cervical os (arrowhead).

FIGURE 10-2 The cervix at 41 weeks of pregnancy. The cervical canal (arrow) shortened and dilated; the amniotic membranes have separated from the lower uterine segment, and the presenting fetal pole, in this case the fetal head covered with vernix(*), is visible. Clinical examination revealed the cervix to be 1 cm in length, 2 to 3 cm dilated, soft, and anteriorly situated.

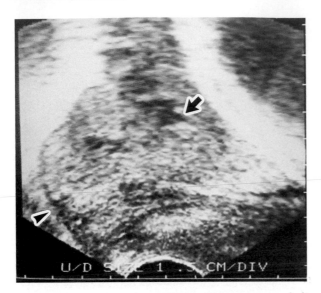

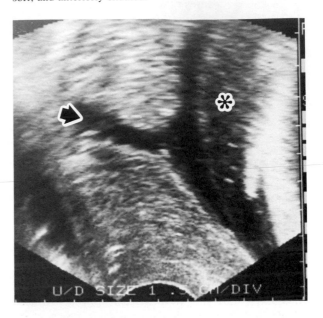

preterm delivery. Even after two preterm deliveries at 20 to 36 weeks, the subsequent term delivery rate exceeds 70% (Bakketeig et al, 1979). Uncertainty regarding clinical criteria for the diagnosis of "cervical incompetence" is reflected in the use of cerclage, since rates among British obstetricians vary between 0% and 8% of all pregnancies (Grant, 1985). Insertion of a cervical suture attempts to prolong pregnancy although there is little evidence of consistent benefit (MRC/RCOG, 1988). Most sutures are placed by the vaginal route in a similar fashion to that described by Shirodkar (1951) or McDonald (1957) with the aim of supporting the internal, cervical os. Abdominal cerclage has been proposed as a more appropriate technique to secure this objective but is less widely used (Novy, 1982). Whether the operation results in substantial benefit has been addressed in the MRC/RCOG multicenter randomized trial of cervical cerclage (MRC/RCOG, 1988). The interim report of this study, detailing the results of 905 patients, suggests "that the operation had an important, beneficial effect in 1 in 20 to 25 cases in the trial. But because the observed differences were not strongly statistically significant and because no such benefit has been seen in other randomized trials, there remains uncertainty about how much (if any) of this apparent benefit is real" (MRC/RCOG, 1988).

FIGURE 10-3 Localization of the inferior border of a low-lying placenta may be achieved with TVS. In this example the lower edge encroaches on the internal cervical os (IO).

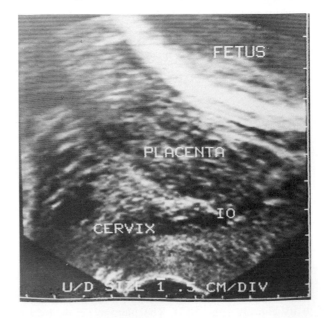

Circlage

Transvaginal sonography (TVS) provides reproducible images of the effects of cervical cerclage. The echogenic material of a circumferential suture is clearly visible in both anterior and posterior lips of the cervix (Fig. 10-4). Vaginal procedures cannot position the suture at, or close to, the internal cervical os, and in most patients the suture is placed in the middle third of the cervix, regardless of the experience of the surgeon (Quinn et al, 1989). Serial scans throughout pregnancy were performed at monthly intervals in a consecutive series of patients undergoing vaginal cerclage. The incidence of cervical cerclage in the study population was less than 0.5% of all pregnancies. Evidence of damage to the internal cervical os, at any stage of pregnancy, was observed in only 2 of 25 patients at 15 and 24 weeks. In both patients the internal cervical os was dilated with concomitant herniation of the gestational sac to the level of the suture (Fig. 10-5). Despite subsequent bed rest in the hospital for the remainder of the pregnancy, preterm delivery occurred at 21 and 32 weeks, respectively. Important features of the damaged internal cervical os associated with cervical incompetence include

FIGURE 10-4 Circumferential Mersilene tape has been inserted by anterior and posterior cervical incisions and appears as a hyperechoic feature in both anterior and posterior lips of the cervix (arrowheads). Cerclage by the vaginal route places the suture in the middle third of the cervical canal. In most patients with a clinical diagnosis of cervical incompetence, the internal cervical os remains closed throughout pregnancy.

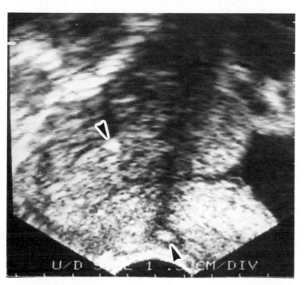

FIGURE 10-5 Cervical incompetence at 16 weeks of pregnancy. The internal cervical os is dilated and irregular with herniation of the gestational sac to the level of the cervical suture (arrowheads). The suture has been inserted in the manner described by Shirodkar and is visible in both anterior and posterior lips of the cervix. The pregnancy aborted at 21 weeks.

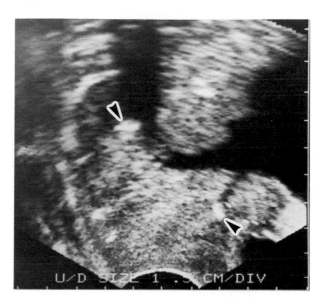

its irregular, asymmetrical dilatation (see Fig. 10-5), in contrast to the symmetrical, smooth appearance associated with decidual resorption over the fetal surface of the internal cervical os that may be a feature of normal pregnancy in the middle trimester (Fig. 10-6). Absence of anatomic damage to the internal cervical os with vaginal scanning does not entirely exclude a diagnosis of cervical incompetence, since that may have occurred in the interval between the scan and the subsequent delivery. In the two patients that such damage was detected, a minimum of 6 weeks elapsed before the subsequent delivery, so it seems unlikely that undetected anatomic damage occurred in the rest of the series. In the overwhelming majority of patients with a clinical diagnosis of cervical incompetence, in a center with a low incidence of the operation, the pregnancy continued to 38 weeks with the internal cervical os closed. The cervical suture was removed, and the pregnancy resulted in successful term delivery.

Cervical cerclage by the vaginal route with subsequent bed rest appears to prolong pregnancy in the rare patient with an anatomic lesion at the internal cervical os. The limited number of patients with this condition appears to preclude a randomized study to identify whether cerclage or cerclage with bed rest is the pre-

FIGURE 10-6 Resorption of the decidua on the fetal surface of the cervix in the region of the internal cervical os at 20 weeks of pregnancy may be mistaken for cervical incompetence. The distinguishing features are the smooth, symmetrical, crescentic appearance that is centered on the internal cervical os (arrow) in contrast to the asymmetrical, irregular appearance of a damaged internal cervical os (see Fig. 10-5).

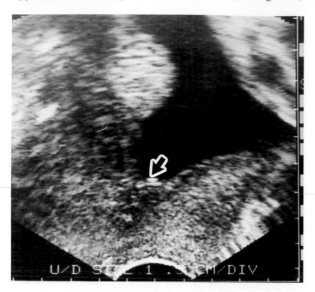

ferred management. The efficacy and position of cerclage by the abdominal route would be of substantial interest in patients with the distinctive anatomic lesion since an improved level of the suture relative to the internal cervical os might be anticipated.

Summary

Potential disadvantages of TVS of the cervix include the biologic effects of ultrasound, the risk of infection, and the release of endogenous prostaglandins. Most endoprobes operate at low power outputs compared with abdominal transducers, although they are closer to the pelvic organs, and reliable in vivo measurements of power exposures have yet to be established. Placing the endoprobe in a sterile disposable glove, together with immersion in glutaraldehyde between patients, constitutes an effective method of avoiding cross-infection.

Finally, given the reduced external dimensions of the endoprobe and the preference of ultrasound scanning over digital vaginal examination of most patients, any release of endogenous prostaglandins may be expected to be less than that of digital vaginal examination. Transperineal scanning is an alternate to TVS of the cervix.

TVS using the appropriate equipment is a safe, patient-acceptable technique for the objective assessment of the cervix throughout pregnancy. Shortening of the cervix and dilation of the cervical canal may be consistently demonstrated. Its role in the management of patients with midtrimester loss associated with cervical incompetence may not represent a major clinical issue in terms of numbers of patients, although reproducible observations regarding the relative positions of sutures and the condition of the internal cervical os may contribute to our understanding of the condition. Whether this technique will help to predict the onset of, or assist in the management of idiopathic preterm labor is an important issue that remains to be addressed.

References

Brown J, Thieme G, Shah D, Fleischer A, Boehm F. Transabdominal and transvaginal sonography: evaluation of the cervix and lower uterine segment. *Am J Obstet Gynecol* 1986;155:721–726.

Bernstine RL, Lee SH, Crawford WL, et al. Sonographic evaluation of the incompetent cervix. *J Clin Ultrasound* 1981;9:417.

Bakketeig LS, Hoffman HJ, Harley EE. The tendency to repeat gestational age and birthweight in successive births. *Am J Obstet Gynecol* 1979;135:1086–1103.

Grant A. MRC/RCOG Randomised Cervical Cerclage Trial Newsletters 1–10. National Perinatal Epidemiology Unit, Oxford. 1985.

Interim Report of the Medical Research Council/Royal College of Obstetricians and Gynaecologists. Multicentre randomised trial of cervical cerclage. *Br J Obstet Gynaecol* 1988;95:437–445.

McDonald IA. Suture of the cervix for inevitable miscarriage. *J Obstet Gynaecol Br Emp* 1957;64:346–350.

Novy MJ. Transabdominal cervicoisthmic cerclage for the management of repetitive abortion and premature delivery. *Am J Obstet Gynecol* 1982;143:44.

Quinn MJ, Farnsworth B, Bisson DL, Stirrat GM. Vaginal ultrasound in the objective assessment of the pregnant cervix. *Br J Radiol* 1989;62:662.

Shirodkar VN. Congress International Jubilaire de La Societe Francais de Gynecologie. Paris, 1951.

Chapter 11

Mid and Late Pregnancy

Bernadette Keefe, MD

Introduction

The second and third trimesters of pregnancy present a different set of diagnostic dilemmas than occur in first-trimester gestation. The problems of ectopic pregnancy and fetal viability are replaced with the issues of fetal anatomy, placental implantation, and cervical competency. Transabdominal sonography (TAS) has been invaluable in clarification of these clinical issues; however, the diagnostic limitations of TAS may be significant in maternal obesity, oligohydramnios, and certain fetal positions. In addition, thorough TAS examination requires an optimally distended urinary bladder, which may distort the status of fetus, placenta, or cervix. Because of these limitations, transvaginal sonography (TVS) is being used in the evaluation of advanced gestation, usually in conjunction with TAS. When the fetus is 13 to 14 weeks gestational age, the transvaginal approach can occasionally be used alone because of the small size of the fetus and uterus at this stage.

The technique of TVS has been well described (Timor-Tritsch et al, 1988). Briefly, TVS is performed with the patient emptying her urinary bladder and lying supine in the dorsal lithotomy position. The transvaginal probe, consisting of a high-frequency transducer at the end of a long handle, is positioned in the mid and proximal vagina. Images of normal and abnormal pelvic structures are obtained in two perpendicular planes. The probe is maneuvered in three basic sagittal planes using elevation and depression, side-to-side, and push/pull motions. Transverse images are obtained by rotating the probe 90 degrees counterclockwise to the sagittal planes. The following points should be noted when TVS is used in the evaluation of the second- and third-trimester gestation. A frequency of 5 MHz is needed by this stage because of the increased sonic range required when evaluating the larger fetus. A higher frequency transducer (6.5 to 7.5 MHz) can be used only if the cervix and the structures close to it are of interest. The probe should be disinfected and covered with a condom and sterile gel to ensure maximal cleanliness. Insertion and positioning of the probe in the vagina should be monitored in real time with documentation of normal midvagina and external and internal cervical os. Such continuous visualization of the vagina and cervix will ensure detection of conditions such as cervical incompetence or vaginal prolapse of amniotic membranes or fetal parts, as well as vaginal masses.

Fetal Anatomy

During TAS, four major factors limit resolution of fetal anatomy: maternal obesity, oligohydramnios, fetal position, and fetal size. In the first instance, fat causes beam scattering resulting in echogenicity on the image. When there is oligohydramnios the normal sonic window (amniotic fluid) is not present, limiting visualization. Also, the fetus moves less, thereby reducing the number of imaging planes.

In the case of a low-lying curled fetus, the extremities may block the sound beam from its ventral surface, and the compressed curved spine is difficult to assess. Finally, early in the second trimester (13 to 15 weeks gestational age), resolution of the small fetal structures may not be possible with the lower frequency transducers used in TAS.

EARLY SECOND TRIMESTER

In many 13- to 14-week gestational age fetuses, a complete obstetric ultrasound examination can be performed using the transvaginal approach. Notably, the effectiveness of TAS is often limited at this stage since a low-frequency transducer is being used to evaluate small fetal structures. With the higher frequency transducer used in TVS these small structures can be detected earlier. At 13 weeks the following fetal structures may be identified with TVS: lateral ventricles and choroid plexus, limbs (including digits), stomach, four-chambered heart, urinary bladder, anterior abdominal wall, spine (only partially developed at this stage), and facial features (Timor-Tritsch et al, 1988). By 13 to 14 weeks the fetal kidneys can be identified. TVS early in the second trimester usually confirms normalcy of the fetus but there is potential for early detection of congenital malformations. Important additional benefits of TVS are that there is no need for a distended urinary bladder and that resolution of structures is not affected by maternal obesity.

Occasionally, TAS may be needed in conjunction with TVS when evaluating the 13- to 14-week pregnancy. This usually occurs when the uterus is extremely anteverted or when the fetus is located high in the fundus. In both of these situations the distance from the transducer to some fetal parts may be less transabdominally than transvaginally. If both TVS and TAS are to be done, the TAS study may be performed with an empty bladder, allowing the fundus to lie closer to the transducer.

MID SECOND TRIMESTER TO TERM

By mid second trimester, most of the fetus lies outside the focal range of the transvaginal probe and TAS is used in diagnosis. Although TVS alone cannot be used in the evaluation of the fetus at this stage, it can be effectively used with TAS in the evaluation of selected fetal structures.

During the 16- to 24-week period, the ultrasonologist is asked to decide whether a gestation is normal or abnormal sonographically. During this time peak α-fetoprotein levels occur, providing a biochemical marker to aid in fetal anomaly detection. Also, fetal structures have increased in size, allowing better detection with ultrasound imaging. At this time therapeutic abortion can be considered if a malformed fetus is found. Unfortunately optimal visualization of major fetal anatomy during the early second trimester is not always possible with TAS (Zador et al, 1988). In such cases a follow-up study is recommended, although this may push diagnosis into the late second trimester, and one cannot always guarantee patient compliance in returning for reevaluation. In addition, increasing maternal weight throughout pregnancy may outweigh the potential benefit of the increasing size and visibility of fetal parts.

When fetal anatomy that is suboptimally evaluated by TAS is located in the lower uterine segment, TVS may be used to great advantage. The vaginal window provides another set of imaging planes at about 90 degrees from those available through TAS. As with TAS, fetal position and movement determine the precise anatomy that TVS can assess. When the fetus is in the cephalic presentation, TVS can be used to evaluate head anatomy, cervical spine, the neck region, and

occasionally the heart, stomach, and anterior abdominal wall (Figs. 11-1 to 11-19). When the fetus is in a breech presentation, the caudal half of the fetus may be visualized by the transvaginal approach; therefore the genitourinary tract, including the kidneys, urinary bladder, genitalia, and potential anomalies thereof can be detected (Figs. 11-5 to 11-8). In these fetuses the fetal stomach, four-chamber heart, and diaphragm may also be in the focal range in the early to mid second trimester. The distal spine is also readily accessible by TVS when the fetus is in the breech lie. The low transverse fetus, often suboptimally evaluated by TAS, may be visualized well by TVS because of the proximity of its entire length to the cervix.

When TAS suggests the presence of a major congenital abnormality but is not definitive, or when there is oligohydramnios with markedly limited resolution, further imaging is done for clarification. In the past amniography and fetoscopy were performed. More recently, investigators reported that computerized tomography (CT) can confirm a suspected diagnosis or add significant information to the TAS study (Siegel et al, 1984). The disadvantage of CT is the radiation to the fetus, which is estimated to be, at maximum, .02 Gy.

Most recently magnetic resonance imaging (MRI) has been used to evaluate suspected abnormal second and third trimester gestations (McCarthy et al, 1985; Fitzmorris-Glass et al, 1989; Williamson et al, 1989). Since motion significantly limits the efficacy of MRI, the fetus must undergo neuromuscular blockade through pancuronium bromide injection in the umbilical vein to ensure fetal immobility. If there is severe oligohydramnios with minimal fetal motion, fetal paralysis may not be necessary. The risks of electromagnetic radiation to the fetus, if any, are unknown. The advantages of MRI include the excellent soft-tissue contrast resolution and detail of the fetal central nervous system and spine obtained.

Although experience using TVS in the older fetus has been limited, TVS promises to have an important ancillary role according to two recent reports (Benacerraf and Estroff, 1989; Bronshtein et al, 1989). Using TVS, Benacerraf and Estroff reported the presence of abnormal cranial anatomy in a second-trimester cephalic fetus; Bronshtein found that TVS better resolved and characterized cystic hygromas in a group of late first- and early second-trimester gestations. In my experience TVS diagnosed renal agenesis associated with caudal regression syndrome when TAS was nondiagnostic.

In summary, transvaginally performed obstetric sonography may be used alone in evaluation of the early second-trimester gestation and in an ancillary role with TAS in older fetuses for evaluation of fetal structures near the cervix. In the latter application TVS can be used to better visualize a suboptimally evaluated fetus or further evaluate a fetal abnormality suspected by the transabdominal study. If there is significant maternal obesity, ancillary TVS is useful, especially if the fetus is in a breech presentation. Also, the breech fetus with oligohydramnios may be evaluated with TVS as the next step after TAS in an attempt to identify the fetal kidneys. TVS evaluation may also enhance examination of presenting twins and the fetus in a low transverse presentation (Fig. 11-9, 11-10). The fetus in cephalic presentation with poorly evaluated cranial anatomy or with a question of hydrocephalus, encephalocoele, or cystic hygroma can be evaluated transvaginally after initial TAS. Such use of adjunctive TVS may be sufficient for diagnosis and obviate the need for more extensive imaging such as CT and MRI.

There are two significant limitations to TVS of advanced gestations. The first is the decreased field of view, causing varying degrees of visualization of the fetus. The second major limitation is the decreased number of scanning planes available from the transvaginal position. This makes the assessment of fetal structures that must be evaluated in precise scanning planes, such as the heart and spine, difficult.

The Cervix

The cervix is an extremely important anatomic and functional structure during pregnancy. Problems with the cervix may seriously affect pregnancy outcome. Ultrasound imaging of the cervix is done mainly to evaluate cervical incompetence and occasionally for the assessment of suspected cervical or cul-de-sac masses (see section on Pelvic Masses). Most experience with cervical sonography has been with the transabdominal full-bladder approach; however, recently there have been reports on the use of TVS to evaluate the status of the cervix.

Cervical incompetence is defined by its classic presentation: painless premature dilation of the cervix with repeated spontaneous abortion in the second trimester. It is considered responsible for 16% to 20% of second-trimester pregnancy loss and up to 25% of preterm deliveries (Parisi, 1988; Michaels et al, 1986). Although the cause of incompetent cervix is multifactorial and not completely understood, there are groups of women known to be at high risk: those with a history of cervical trauma (especially dilation and curettage, therapeutic abortion, traumatic delivery, and cervical conization) and those with congenital abnormalities of the genital tract (Shortle and Jewelewicz, 1989). The incidence ranges from 0.2% to 2%. The standard for diagnosis is the physical examination that reveals cervical effacement, shortening, or dilation. Limitations of the physical examination include its dependency on the

experience of the examiner, interexaminer variability, and the fact that some mild cervical dilation is common during the late second trimester (Parisi, 1988).

In an effort to increase diagnostic accuracy in assessing cervical incompetence, sonography using the transabdominal full bladder approach, has been used. The chief limitation of this technique has been the adverse effect of the distended urinary bladder (Confino et al, 1986). When distended, the urinary bladder applies direct pressure to the lower uterine segment and cervix, causing the cervix to appear lengthened. Such pressure can also compress an open cervical canal, thereby masking cervical incompetence. Other limitations of TAS include poor visualization of the cervix in low cephalic presentations due to attenuation of the sound beam by the fetal head, and inaccurate measurement of cervical length due to limited resolution of the endocervical canal. Nonetheless, cervical incompetence can be adequately demonstrated by TAS, with signs varying from the small nipple of early cervical protrusion to frank herniation with hourglass membranes. Despite the limitations of TAS in evaluating the status of the cervix, the following observations have been made (Ayers et al, 1988; Feingold et al, 1984; Ludmir, 1988; Parisi, 1988; Podobnik et al, 1988; Varma et al, 1986).

1. Longitudinal cervical length measurements vary from 2.5 to 5.0 cm in healthy pregnancies and 2.0 to 4.0 cm in cases of incompetent cervix. The potential for overlap of normal and abnormal cervical measurements appears less within an ultrasound facility than between facilities. Also, each patient can serve as her own control, whereby shortening of the cervix between scans would be suggestive of cervical incompetence.

2. Widening of the cervical canal with resultant increase in diameter of the internal cervical os is also important in diagnosing cervical incompetence. An internal os width of greater than 1.9 cm and endocervical canal width of greater than 6 mm are associated with incompetence. The cervix is by definition incompetent if herniated membrane or fetal parts are visualized in the endocervical canal.

3. Serial cervical sonography in high-risk patients may detect the incompetent cervix before the obstetrician's physical examination.

4. Preterm uterine activity, vaginal bleeding, and cervical length shortening are associated with the risk of premature delivery. Additionally, it is not known whether premature cervical length shortening is an effect of preterm labor or a symptom of cervical incompetence; therefore the clinical and sonographic findings must be considered together.

5. Cervical incompetence is a dynamic process evaluated at short intervals (usually weekly) by both

physical examination and sonography. Rapidly progressive incompetence may be detected late by both methods (Brown et al, 1986).

TVS can increase the accuracy of cervical sonography because with TVS there is no cervical distortion from the urinary bladder distention or external transducer pressure.There also are no intervening structures to cause attenuation of the sound beam. Inaccurate measurement of the cervical canal is also less of a problem with TVS because the increased resolution of the images permits excellent delineation of the entire length of the endocervical canal (Figs. 11-11, 11-12). It is notable that in one study where TVS was compared with TAS in evaluation of the cervix, measurements of the cervix were more easily obtained and more reproducible with TVS than with full-bladder TAS (Brown et al, 1986).

To date there is limited experience with transvaginally obtained cervical length measurements (Fig. 11–20). Guidelines for the use of TVS in detecting cervical incompetence include establishment of normal cervical measurements in pregnant patients; obtaining baseline cervical measurement of high risk patients in the late first trimester; and performance of serial scans at frequent regular intervals with correlation to the physical examination. A baseline cervical length measurement considered shorter than the norm seen in the ultrasound facility, a decrease in the cervical length from baseline ultrasound studies, an internal os diameter of greater than 1.9 cm, or an endocervical canal diameter greater than 6 mm suggest cervical incompetence.

Treatments for cervical incompetence vary from bed rest in the Trendelenburg position to cervical cerclage. The placement of a cervical suture in select patients is thought to prolong pregnancy and have a fetal salvage rate of 58% to 77%. Sonography has been used to evaluate both the Shirodkar and the McDonald cerclage techniques (Parulekar and Kiwi, 1982). Parulekar and Kiwi found that the 5 mm Mersilene tape used in the Shirodkar technique was better visualized than McDonald's No. 2 nylon suture. On average, the tape was seen at 2.4 cm from the external os, whereas the suture was seen at 1.5 cm. Sonography can be helpful in the follow-up of patients after cerclage to assess the possibility of membrane herniation beyond the level of cerclage.

Placenta Previa

Placenta previa is the abnormal location of the placenta in the lower uterine segment. The incidence at term is 0.6% (Naeye, 1978). The relationship of the placental edge to the internal cervical os is vital information for the obstetrician. The most significant risks are maternal hemorrhage and increased perinatal mortality (McShane et al, 1985). Terms used to describe the severity of the condition include low-lying placenta (placental location in the lower uterine segment but not on the cervix), marginal previa (when the placental edge is located on the ipsilateral cervical lip), partial previa (when the edge of the placenta covers a small portion of the internal os), and complete previa (when the bulk of the placenta overlies the cervical os) (Pritchard et al, 1985). There is an increased incidence of placenta previa in patients with histories of caesarean section, dilation and curettage, spontaneous abortion, and evacuation of retained products of conception, suggesting damage to the endometrium and myometrium as possible causes (Rose and Chapman, 1986).

The first diagnosis of placenta previa using TAS was in 1966. Since that time full-bladder TAS has been the mainstay for diagnosis. The lowest reported false-positive and false-negative rates for the diagnosis of placenta previa using TAS and 2% each (Laing, 1981; Bowie et al, 1978). Factors that decrease visibility during TAS include maternal obesity and attenuation of the ultrasound beam by the fetal cranium (Fig. 11–13). With TAS the low posterior placenta is difficult to evaluate. The most significant drawback to TAS is the necessity of a distended urinary bladder, which frequently causes distortion of the lower uterine segment and a false diagnosis of placenta previa, particularly when the placenta is located along the anterior wall of the lower uterine segment, (Bowie et al, 1983; Townsend et al, 1986; Zemlyn, 1978). Techniques to circumvent such limitations have included Trendelenburg positioning, fetal elevation, and pre- and postvoid bladder imaging (Artis et al, 1985; Jeffrey and Laing, 1981; Lee et al, 1981). It is also now recognized that most of the false positive diagnoses of placenta previa made in midtrimester evaluations resulted from the differential growth between the uterus and placenta, which causes the change in the placenta/os relationship seen at term. For this reason rescanning in the late third trimester is recommended to confirm the diagnosis (Gallagher et al, 1987). MRI has been used to evaluate cases of suspected previa with good results (Powell et al, 1986). The location of the placenta with respect to the cervical os can be determined using T2-weighted spin-echo sequences in the sagittal plane.

Recently, sonography using the vaginal approach has been performed to evaluate the possibility of placenta previa (Farine et al, 1988; Farine et al, 1989). TVS is not limited by the factors that inhibit the transabdominal examination—maternal obesity, distended urinary bladder, obstructing fetal parts, or posterior implantation of the placenta (Fig. 11-14 to 11-16, 11-21). Additionally, TVS uses a higher frequency transducer (less depth penetration is required), resulting in higher resolution images. Although vaginal manipulation is usually contraindicated in suspected previa, in the largest series (55 patients examined), there was no evidence of vaginal bleeding up to 24 hours after TVS (Powel et al, 1986). In this report, Farine and colleagues also emphasized that for optimal imaging the probe tip should be placed several centimeters from the cervix. These investigators were able to identify the internal cervical os in 100% of cases using TVS but only in 65% using TAS. Using TVS they made the correct diagnosis in 87% of patients with suspected placenta previa, but when using TAS they were correct in less than half the cases. They also recommend rescanning at term because of the high false-positive rate when scanning in the second trimester.

Miscellaneous Applications

PELVIC MASSES IN PREGNANCY

Pelvis masses are detected frequently in pregnancy through physical examination and, in most cases, do not cause complications. When the organ of origin and size and cause of the mass are of concern, or if the patient is symptomatic, ultrasound imaging is used for further evaluation.

Uterine myoma is the most common pelvic mass in pregnancy, it has an incidence of 0.3% to 2.6%. Up to 10% of myomas will grow in pregnancy (Bezjian, 1984). Masses of ovarian origin are the second most common type of pelvic mass in pregnancy. The most common of these is the corpus luteum cyst. The corpus luteum cyst is usually a simple cyst, measuring less than 4 cm, which regresses by 16 weeks gestation. These cysts may become symptomatic when hemorrhagic or if they undergo torsion, however. The most frequently occurring complex cystic ovarian mass in pregnancy is a dermoid (Bezjian, 1984). Solid ovarian masses are rare. There is a 3% to 5% incidence of malignancy in ovarian masses during pregnancy. Sonography is used to confirm the presence of a pelvic mass, to determine the organ of origin (usually uterine or ovarian), and to characterize the echotextural features of the lesion to formulate a differential diagnosis. Sonography is also used to follow a mass to resolution, to establish its persistence, or to document a change in size.

Using TVS, one can usually diagnose uterine fibroids, which are typically solid. A fibroid located in the lower uterine segment or cervical region may not be well visualized with TAS, however. This is especially true in maternal obesity and after the first trimester when the growing fetus may cause attenuation of the ultrasound beam. Additionally, if the fibroid has under-

gone cystic degeneration, it may resemble a cystic ovarian mass. With maternal obesity, the increased gain needed for the ultrasonic beam to penetrate may cause a cystic ovarian mass to appear solid. When masses are located deep in the pelvis and in the region of the cul-de-sac, it is often impossible to determine whether the lesion is uterine or ovarian in origin using TAS.

When TAS is limited by maternal habitus or location of the mass, TVS may be useful (Fleischer et al, 1989; Lande et al, 1988; Leibman et al, 1988; Mendelson et al, 1988; Tessler et al, 1989). Pelvic masses in proximity to the transvaginal probe tip include myoma of the lower uterine segment or cervix, ovarian mass, bicornuate uterus, and retroverted uterus (Figs. 11-17, 11-18). In most cases TVS can determine whether the lesion is uterine or ovarian despite confounding echotextural characteristics. When the mass is large, however, TAS may be needed in addition to TVS. After the third or fourth month of gestation, the ovaries are located out of the true pelvis and thus not visible transvaginally. In these situations, and in evaluation of the body and fundus of the uterus, TAS and sometimes MRI can be performed.

TRANSVAGINAL DOPPLER IN PREGNANCY

TVS has been used for Doppler evaluation of uterine and fetal vessels. An initial report demonstrated the use of a transvaginal probe equipped with a radiating sector transducer containing a pulsed and gated Doppler beam to evaluate the uterine arteries in the parametrium (Deutinger et al, 1988). Advantages of this approach were direct visualization of the uterine artery and bilateral sampling. In another report, transvaginal pulsed Doppler was used to evaluate fetal arteries (Deutinger et al, 1989). In this case the authors demonstrated the advantage of the transvaginal approach over the transabdominal method when evaluating fetal arteries in settings of maternal obesity, hydramnios, difficult umbilical cord presentation, and low-lying cephalic presentations.

Summary

In conclusion, TVS has a definite role in the evaluation of the advanced gestation, and there is the promise of expanded indications in the future. When the fetal anatomy, distal placenta, and cervical os are not optimally visualized by TAS, TVS may be useful. Also TVS may be used to evaluate pelvic masses that are located deep in the pelvis. In certain patients, the transvaginal approach is preferable to the transabdominal route when performing obstetrical Doppler. In general, TVS can contribute to the evaluation of maternal and fetal structures located in the true pelvis regardless of the gestational age of the pregnancy.

References

Artis AA III, Bowie JD, Rosenberg ER, Rauch RF. The fallacy of placental migration: effect of sonographic techniques. *AJR* 1985;144:79–81.

Ayers JWT, DeGrood RM, Compton AA, Barclay M, Ansbacher R. Sonographic evaluation of cervical length in pregnancy: diagnosis and management of preterm cervical effacement in patients at risk for premature delivery. *Obstet Gynecol* 1988;71:939–944.

Benacerraf BR, Estroff JA. Transvaginal sonographic imaging of the low fetal head in the second trimester. *J Ultrasound Med* 1989;8:325–328.

Bezjian AA. Pelvic masses in pregnancy. *Clin Obstet Gynecol* 1984;27:402–415.

Bowie JD, Rochester D, Cadkin AV, et al. Accuracy of placental localization by ultrasound. *Radiology* 1978; 128:177–180.

Bowie JD, Andreotti RF, Rosenberg ER. Sonographic appearance of the uterine cervix in pregnancy: the vertical cervix. *AJR* 1983;140:737–740.

Bronshtein M, Rottem S, Yoffe N, Blumenfeld Z. First-trimester and early second-trimester diagnosis of nuchal cystic hygroma by transvaginal sonography: diverse prognosis of the septated from the nonseptated lesion. *Am J Obstet Gynecol* 1989;161:78–82.

Brown JE, Thieme GA, Shah DM, Fleischer AC, Boehm FH. Transabdominal and transvaginal endosonography: evaluation of the cervix and lower uterine segment in pregnancy. *Am J Obstet Gynecol* 1986;155:721–726.

Confino E, Mayden KL, Giglia RV, Vermesh M, Gleicher N. Pitfalls in sonographic imaging of the incompetent uterine cervix. *Acta Obstet Gynecol Scand* 1986;65:593–597.

Deutinger J, Rudelstorfer R, Bernaschek G. Vaginosonographic velocimetry of both main uterine arteries by visual vessel recognition and pulsed Doppler method during pregnancy. *Am J Obstet Gynecol* 1988;159:1072–1076.

Deutinger J, Rudelstorfer R, Hausler P, Bernaschek G. Transvaginal pulsed Doppler velocimetry in fetal arteries. *Arch Gynecol Obstet* 1989;246:57–60.

Farine D, Fox HE, Jakobson S, Timor-Tritsch IE. Vaginal ultrasound for diagnosis of placenta previa. *Am J Obstet Gynecol* 1988;159:566–569.

Farine D, Fox HE, Jakobson S, Timor-Tritsch IE. Is it really a placenta previa? *Eur J Obstet Gynecol* 1989;31:103–108.

Feingold M, Brook I, Zakut H. Detection of cervical incompetence by ultrasound. *Acta Obstet Gynecol Scand* 1984;63:407–410.

Fitzmorris-Glass R, Mattrey RF, Cantrell CJ. Magnetic resonance imaging as an adjunct to ultrasound in oligohydramnios: detection of sirenomelia. *J Ultrasound Med* 1989;8:159–162.

Fleischer AC, Gordon AN, Entman SS. Transabdominal and transvaginal sonography of pelvic masses. *Ultrasound Med Biol* 1989;15:529–533.

Gallagher P, Fagan CJ, Bedi DG, Winsett MZ, Reyes RN. Potential placenta previa: definition, frequency, and significance. *AJR* 1987;149:1013–1015.

Gottesfeld KR, Thompson IIE, Holmes JH, Taylor ES. Ultrasonic placentography: a new method for placental localization. *Am J Obstet Gynecol* 1966;96:538–546.

Jeffrey RB, Laing FC. Sonography of the low-lying placenta: value of trendelenburg and traction scans. *AJR* 1981;137:547–549.

Laing FC. Placenta previa: avoiding false-negative diagnoses. *J Clin Ultrasound* 1981;9:109–113.

Lande IM, Hill MC, Cosco FE, Kator NN. Adnexal and cul-de-sac abnormalities: transvaginal sonography. *Radiology* 1988;166:325–332.

Lee TG, Knochel JQ, Melendez MG, Henderson SC. Fetal elevation: a new technique for placental localization in the diagnosis of previa. *Clin Ultrasound* 1981;9:467–471.

Leibman AJ, Kruse B, McSweeney MB. Transvaginal sonography: comparison with transabdominal sonography in the diagnosis of pelvic masses. *AJR* 1988;151:89–92.

Ludmir J. Sonographic detection of cervical incompetence. *Clin Obstet Gynecol* 1988;31:101–109.

McCarthy SM, Filly RA, Stark DD, et al. Magnetic resonance imaging of fetal anomalies in utero: early experience. *AJR* 1985;145:677–682.

McShane PM, Heyl PS, Epstein MF. Maternal and perinatal morbidity resulting from placenta previa. *Obstet Gynecol* 1985;65:176–182.

Mendelson EB, Bohm-Velez M, Neiman HL, Russo J. Transvaginal sonography in gynecologic imaging. *Semin US, CT, MR* 1988;9:102–121.

Michaels WH, Montgomery C, Karo J, et al. Ultrasound differentiation of the competent from the incompetent cervix: prevention of preterm delivery. *Am J Obstet Gynecol* 1986;154:537–546.

Naeye RL. Placenta praevia: predisposing factors and effects on the fetus and surviving infants. *Obstet Gynecol* 1978;52:521–528.

Parisi VM. Cervical incompetence and preterm labor. *Clin Obstet Gynecol* 1988;31:585–598.

Parulekar SG, Kiwi R. Ultrasound evaluation of sutures following cervical cerclage for incompetent cervix uteri. *J Ultrasound Med* 1982;1:223–228.

Podobnik M, Bulic M, Smiljanic N, Bistricki J. Ultrasonography in the detection of cervical incompetency. *J Clin Ultrasound* 1988;13:383–391.

Powel MC, Buckley J, Price H, Worthington BS, Symonds EM. Magnetic resonance imaging and placenta previa. *Am J Obstet Gynecol* 1986; 154:565–569.

Pritchard JA, MacDonald PC, Grant NF. *Williams Obstetrics*, 17th ed. Norwalk: Appleton-Century Crofts. 1985;976.

Rose GL, Chapman MG. Aetiological factors in placenta praevia: a case controlled study. *Br J Obstet Gynaecol* 1986;93:586–588.

Shortle B, Jewelewicz R. Cervical incompetence. *Fertil Steril* 1989;52:181–188.

Siegel HA, Seltzer SE, Miller S. Prenatal computed tomography: are there indications? *J Comput Assist Tomogr* 1984;8:871–876.

Tessler FN, Schiller VL, Perella RR, Sutherland ML, Grant EG. Transabdominal versus endovaginal pelvic sonography: prospective study. *Radiology* 1989;170:553–556.

Timor-Tritsch IE, Rottem S, Elgali S. How transvaginal sonography is done. In: Timor-Tritsch IE, Rottem S, eds. *Transvaginal Sonography*. New York: Elsevier Science, 1988:109–124.

Townsend RR, Laing FC, Nyberg DA, Jeffrey RB, Wing VW. Technical factors responsible for "placental migration": sonographic assessment. *Radiology* 1986;160:105–108.

Varma TR, Patel RH, Pillai U. Ultrasonic assessment of cervix in "at risk" patients. *Acta Obstet Gynecol Scand* 1986; 65:147–152.

Weinreb JC, Brown CE, Lowe TW, Cohen JM, Erdman WA. Pelvic masses in pregnant patients: MR and US imaging. *Radiology* 1986;159:717–724.

Williamson RA, Weiner CP, Yuh WTC, Abu-Yousef MM. Magnetic resonance imaging of anomalous fetuses. *Obstet Gynecol* 1989;73:952–956.

Witter FR. Negative sonographic findings followed by rapid cervical dilatation due to cervical incompetence. *Obstet Gynecol* 1984; 64:136–137.

Zador IE, Bottoms SF, Tse GM, Brindley BA, Sokol RJ. Nomograms for ultrasound visualization of fetal organs. *J Ultrasound Med* 1988;7:197–201.

Zemlyn S. The effect of the urinary bladder in obstetrical sonography. *Radiology* 1978;128:169–175.

FIGURE 11-1   TAS provides a limited evaluation of the cranial contents because of marked attenuation of the ultrasound beam by the fetal skull (gestational age: 36 weeks).

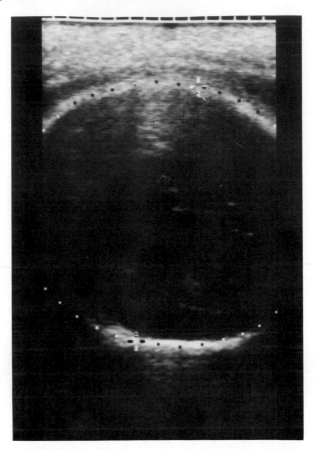

FIGURE 11-2   TVS in same patient as Figure 11-1 demonstrates in detail the fetal head in a coronal plane. The improved resolution is largely due to the use of a high-frequency transducer and the use of the anterior fontanelle as an ultrasonic window. The images show mild to moderate dilation of the frontal horns.

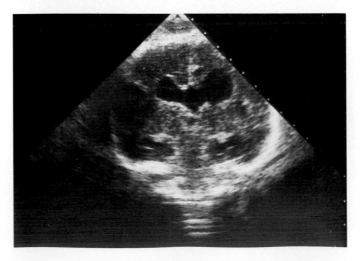

FIGURE 11-3   TAS of the lower uterine segment shows poor definition of the fetal head, seen here to abut the cervix (gestational age: 18 weeks).

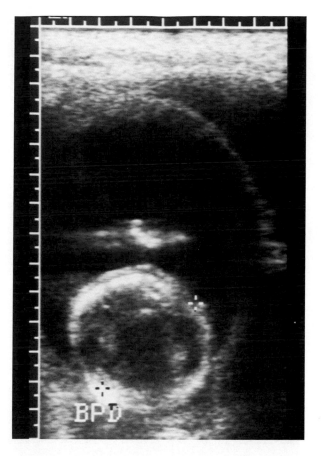

FIGURE 11-4   TVS in the same patient as Figure 11-3 reveals the normal cranial anatomy expected at this gestational age. Symmetric choroid plexi and lateral ventricles are demonstrated.

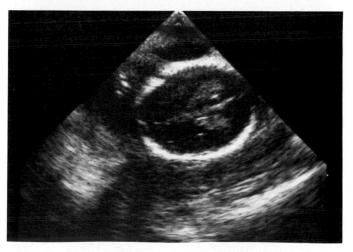

FIGURE 11-5   TAS (two separate images) in this low-lying, curled, breech fetus is limited. Evaluation of the ventral aspect of the fetus is especially suboptimal (gestational age: 16 weeks).

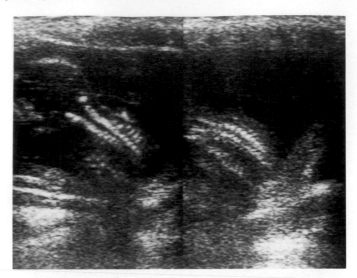

FIGURE 11-6   TVS in the same patient as Figure 11-5 shows the entrance of the umbilical vessels (arrow) into the fetal abdomen.

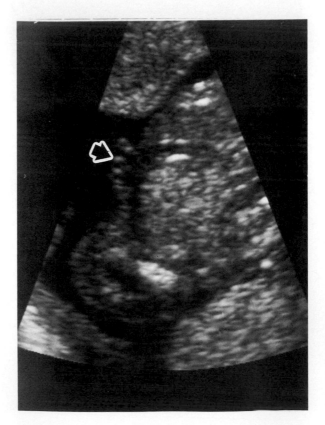

FIGURE 11-7 TAS (two images) in this obese mother (weighing almost 300 pounds) is severely limited and, except for obtaining fetal measurements, is not diagnostic. The fetus is breech (gestational age: 15 weeks).

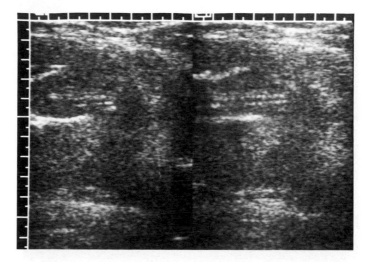

FIGURE 11-8 TVS in the same patient as Figure 11-7 shows both kidneys just lateral to the spine in this coronal view. A normal distal spine and urinary bladder could also be seen using TVS.

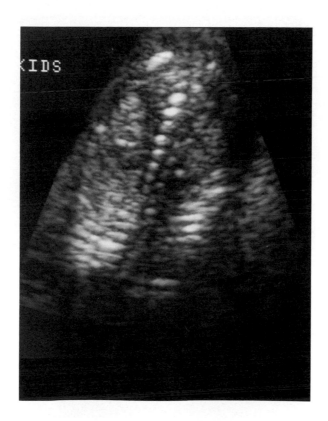

FIGURE 11-9   TAS (in this twin gestation) demonstrates twin A in a low, curled, breech presentation. The fetal anatomy could not be well visualized because of the difficult presentation (gestational age: 18 weeks). Twin B, not pictured here, was situated in the fundus and well visualized with TAS.

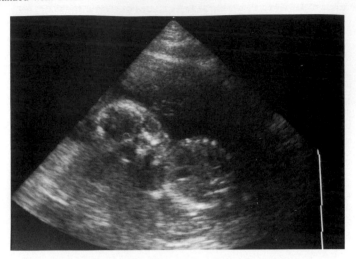

FIGURE 11-10   TVS of twin A seen in Figure 11-9 shows the normal four-chambered heart, not possible to demonstrate with TAS. Symmetric atria and ventricles are well delineated.

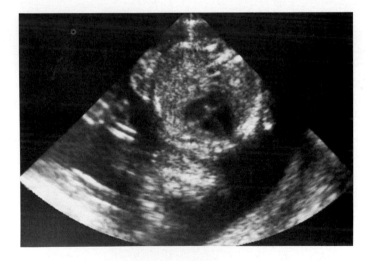

Mid and Late Pregnancy

FIGURE 11-11 TVS in the sagittal plane demonstrates a normal cervix in this term pregnancy. The edges of the internal os are approximated. The fetal head abuts the cervix.

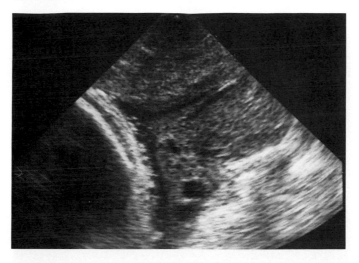

FIGURE 11-12 TVS in the sagittal plane demonstrates "funneling" of the endocervical canal caused by herniation of fetal membranes into the proximal portion of the endocervical canal.

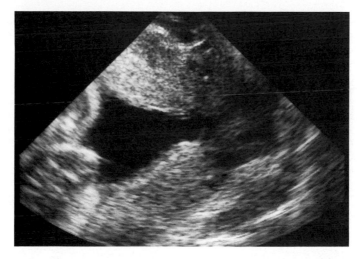

FIGURE 11-13 TAS (2 images) of the lower uterine segment (in the saggital plane) is limited because of maternal obesity (gestational age: 14 weeks).

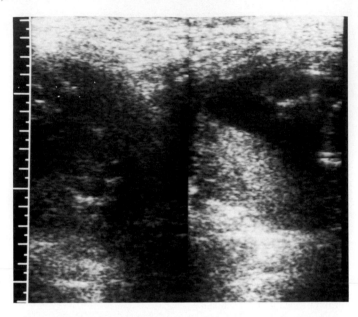

FIGURE 11-14 TVS performed after TAS shown in Figure 11-13 demonstrates the normal internal cervical os and a low-lying placenta implanted close to but not on the cervix (saggital plane).

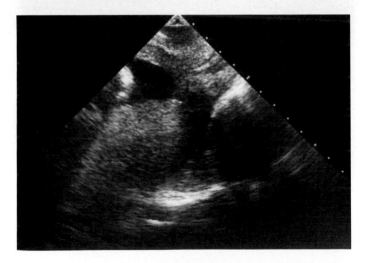

FIGURE 11-15   TVS in the sagittal plane shows a posterior placenta with partial placenta previa (gestational age: 29 weeks).

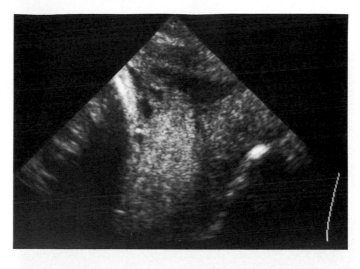

FIGURE 11-16   TVS of the cervix in the sagittal plane shows complete placenta previa (* = placenta; gestational age: 19 weeks).

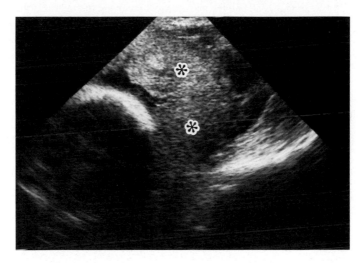

FIGURE 11-17   TVS of the cervical region in the sagittal plane demonstrates a large cervical fibroid (between cursor) posterior to the cervical canal (arrow). With the additional resolution afforded by TVS, we would correctly determine the uterine origin of this mass in the cul-de-sac. The diagnosis could not be made using TAS (gestational age: 18 weeks).

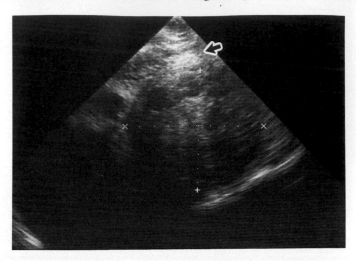

FIGURE 11-18   TVS of the right adnexa shows a complex mass (arrow) involving the right ovary in this patient suspected of having a right ectopic pregnancy. A normal intrauterine fetus, not pictured here, was demonstrated with TVS (gestational age: 13 weeks).

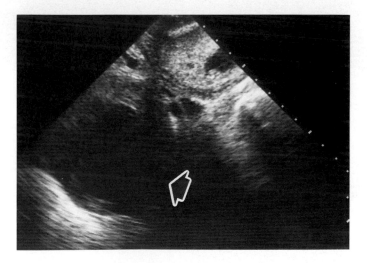

FIGURE 11-19   **Fetal Abnormalities**

11-19A   A TVS of an ancephalic 14-week fetus.

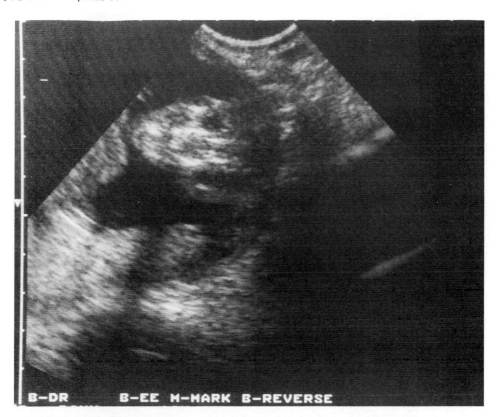

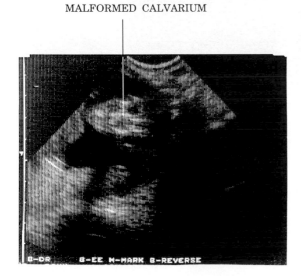

MALFORMED CALVARIUM

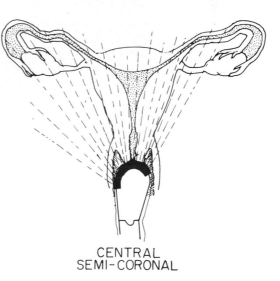

CENTRAL
SEMI-CORONAL

(continued)

FIGURE 11-19   **Fetal Abnormalities** *(continued)*

11-19B   TVS of cojoined twins with two heads.

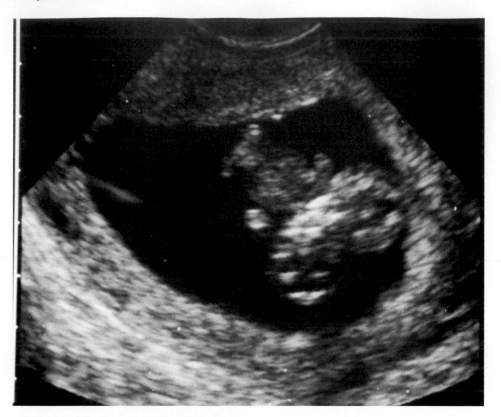

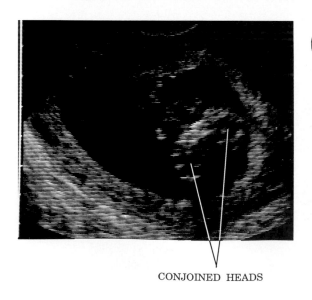

CONJOINED HEADS

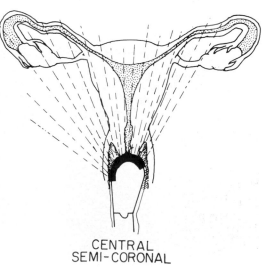

CENTRAL
SEMI-CORONAL

FIGURE 11-20   Normal Cervix

11-20A   TVS of normal gravid cervix in long axis during second trimester.

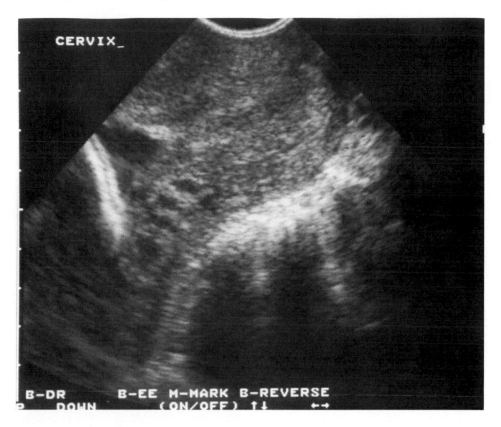

INTERNAL OS   EXTERNAL OS

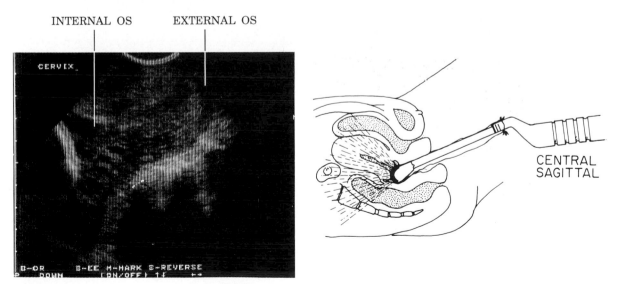

CENTRAL SAGITTAL

(continued)

FIGURE 11-20   Normal Cervix *(continued)*

11-20B   Transperineal sonogram of normal gravid cervix during third trimester.

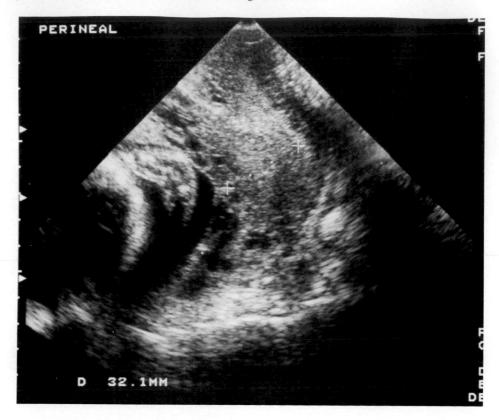

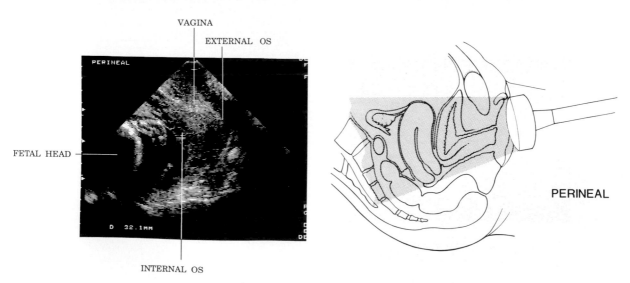

FIGURE 11-21   TVS of placenta previa with retroplacental hemorrhage.

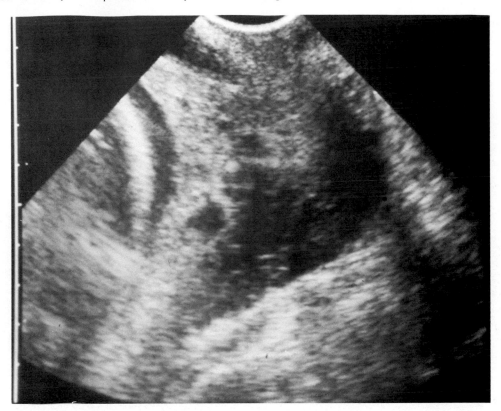

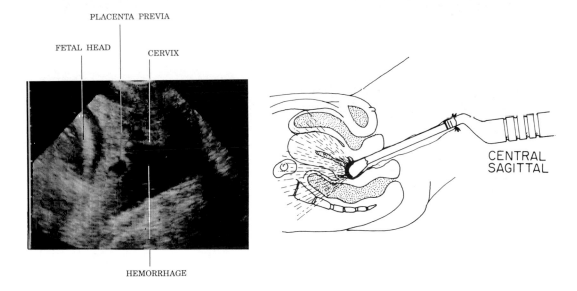

PLACENTA PREVIA

FETAL HEAD

CERVIX

CENTRAL
SAGITTAL

HEMORRHAGE

FIGURE 11-22 Transvaginal sonogram of 13-week fetus with a cystic hygroma.

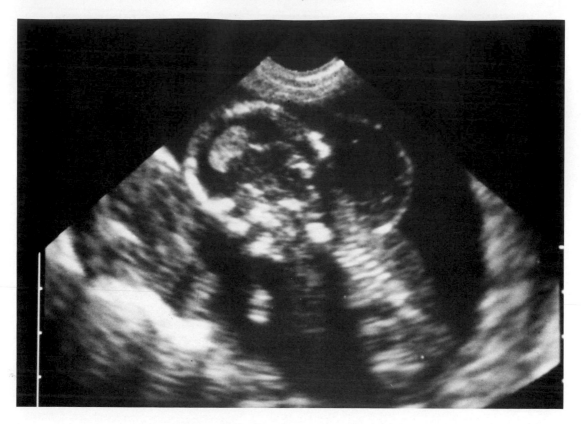

CYSTIC HYGROMA

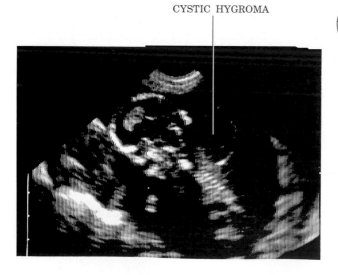

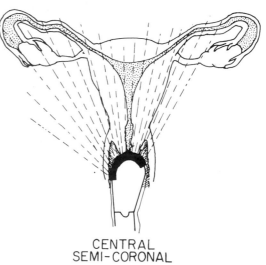

CENTRAL
SEMI-CORONAL

FIGURE 12-1 Normal Uterine Vessels

12-1A Triplex TV CDS showing main uterine artery (blue). There is moderate diastolic flow in this scan done in the late proliferative phase.

12-1B Triplex TV CDS showing arcuate arteries (red) coursing within the outer myometrium.

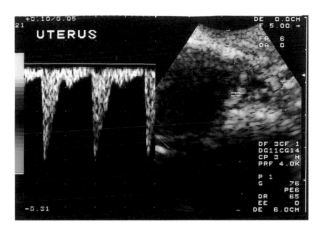

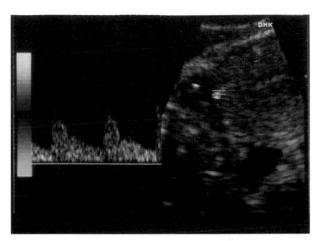

12-1C Triplex TV CDS demonstrating arcuate veins (blue). Waveform shows minor respiratory variation.

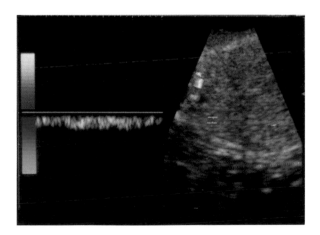

(continued)

FIGURE 12-1 Normal Uterine Vessels *(continued)*

12-1D Radial vessels seen branching from arcuate coursing toward endometrium.

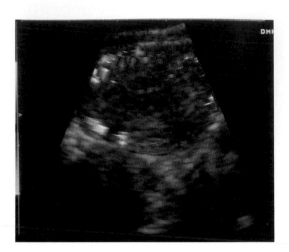

12-1E Normal uterine arcuate arterial flow in 5-week intrauterine pregnancy. Increased flow within the arcuate vessels is readily seen. Only limited flow within the choriodecidua is present.

12-1F Venous flow within choriodecidua of same 5-week intrauterine pregnancy as shown in *E*.

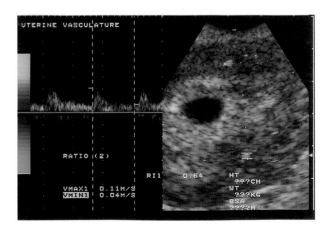

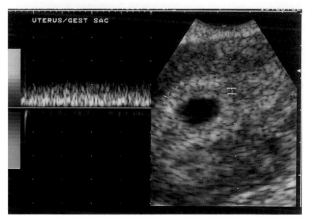

FIGURE 12-2   **Normal Ovarian Vessels**

12-2A   Triplex TV CDS showing no diastolic flow in vessels surrounding two immature follicles.

12-2B   Same patient as *A* in the postovulatory phase showing significant diastolic flow within wall of corpus luteum.

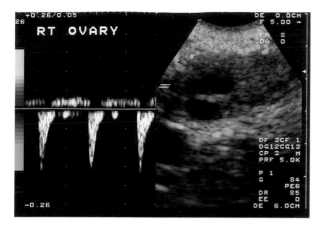 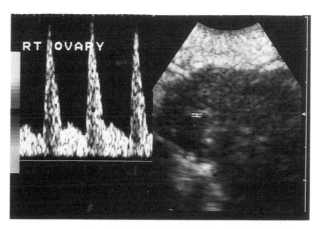

12-2C, D   Triplex image of left ovary containing a mature follicle showing arterial (*C*) and venous (*D*) flow.

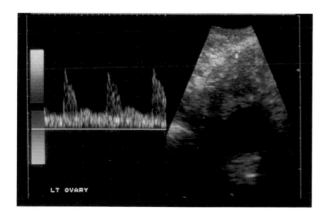 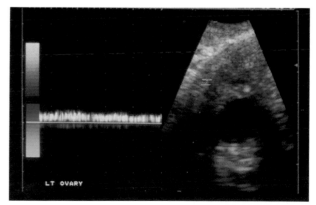

(continued)

FIGURE 12-2 Normal Ovarian Vessels *(continued)*

12-2E Triplex TV CDS showing arterial waveform arising from adnexal branch of uterine artery coursing toward the right ovary.

12-2F Triplex TV CDS of adnexal branch of uterine artery supplying right ovary.

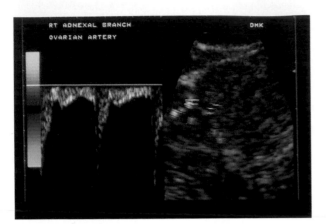

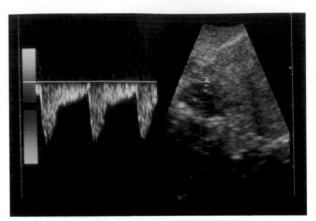

12-2G Triplex TV CDS of an arcuate uterine vein.

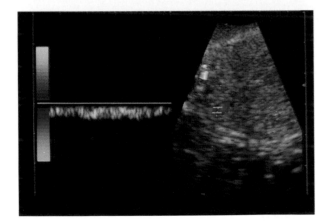

FIGURE 12-3 Uterine Disorders

12-3A Arterial waveform from cervical ectopic pregnancy 1 day after first dose of methotrexate therapy.

12-3B Venous waveform from cervical ectopic pregnancy 1 day after first dose of methotrexate therapy.

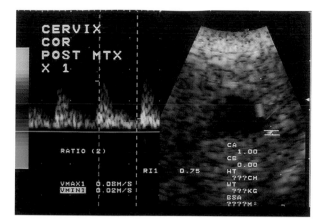

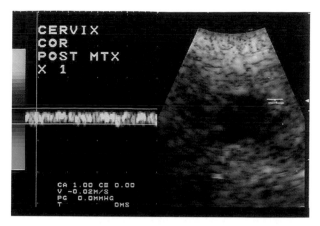

12-3C Same patient as *A* and *B* after four doses of methotrexate demonstrating slightly decreased maximum systolic arterial velocities.

12-3D Same patient as *C* showing decreased venous velocities as well.

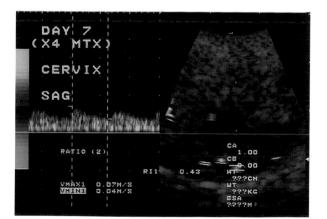

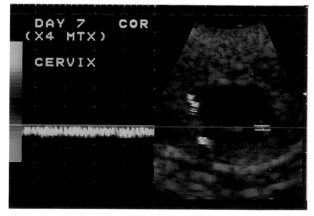

(continued)

FIGURE 12-3 Uterine Disorders *(continued)*

12-3E TV CDS showing vessels surrounding twin intrauterine pregnancy at 6 weeks in a patient with bleeding.

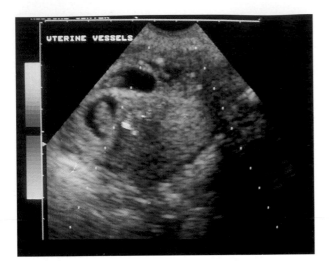

12-3F TV CDS in patient with bicornuate uterus and an intrauterine pregnancy at 9 weeks demonstrating vessels surrounding choriodecidua.

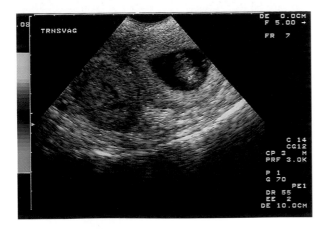

FIGURE 12-4 Ovarian Masses

12-4A Ovarian cyst showing no diastolic flow.

12-4B Hemorrhagic ovarian cyst demonstrating typical "notched" diastolic flow and hemorrhage within cyst.

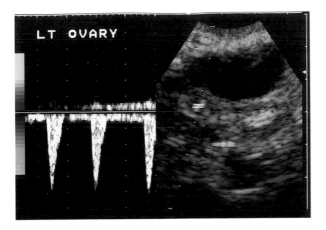

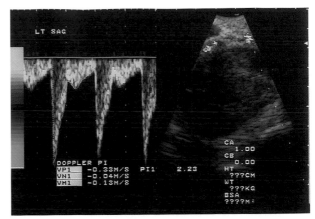

12-4C Endometrioma demonstrating different waveforms. In area surrounding ovary, there is no diastolic flow.

12-4D Endometrioma shown in C demonstrating different waveforms. Vessels within the wall show a low PI. At surgery, extensive vascularity within the peritoneum was seen at this site.

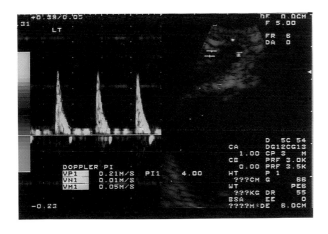

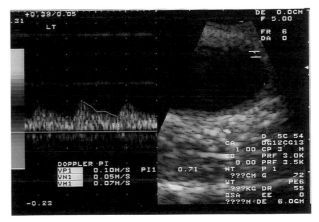

(continued)

FIGURE 12-4 Ovarian Masses *(continued)*

12-4E Multiloculated serous cystadenocarcinoma with flow in area of thick septation. Low PI indicative of tumor.

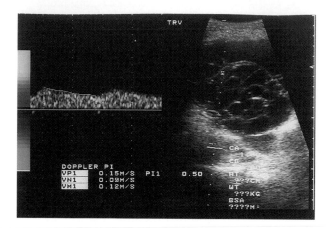

12-4F Central venous flow in same areas as *E*.

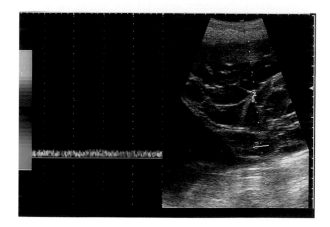

12-4G, H Arterial and venous flow within solid area of an immature teratoma with a low PI similar to that seen in malignant tumors.

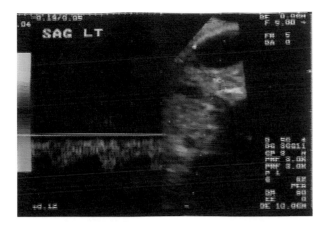
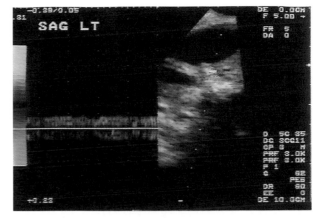

12-4I Solid ovarian mass with cystic areas. The arterial branches have a low PI. This represented a papillary serous cystadenocarcinoma.

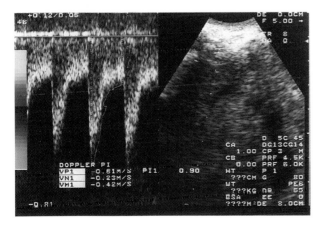

FIGURE 12-5 Ovulation Induction

12-5A Venous flow in patient undergoing Perganol ovulation induction.

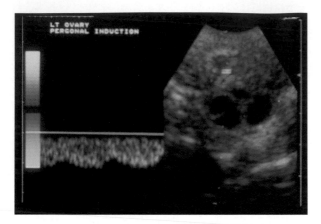

12-5B Same patient as in *A* 6 days later demonstrating enlargement of follicles and venous flow within ovary, thus excluding torsion.

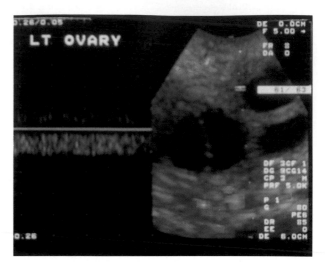

12-5C Low resistance, high diastolic arterial flow in a hyperstimulated ovary.

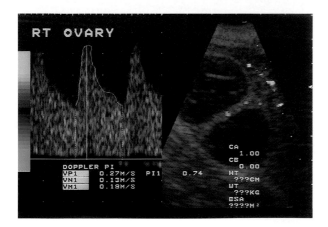

FIGURE 12-6   Other Conditions

12-6A   Ovarian torsion. Enlarged ovary with no flow distal to pedicle.

12-6B   Dilated veins surrounding ovary in patient with pelvic congestion syndrome.

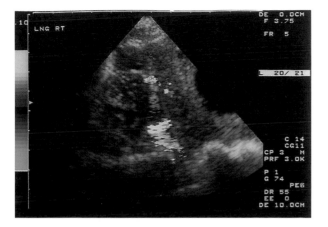

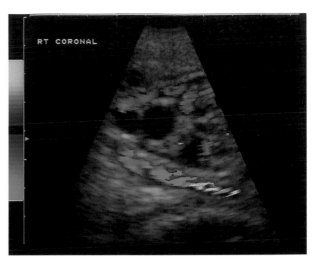

12-6C   Dilated uterine veins in a patient with pelvic congestion syndrome.

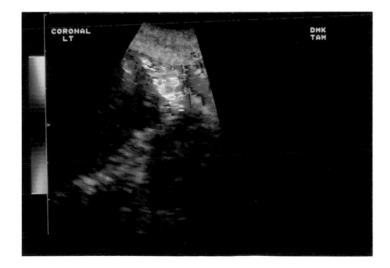

FIGURE 12-7 Placenta accreta. Flow within vessels that invaded the myometrium is shown.

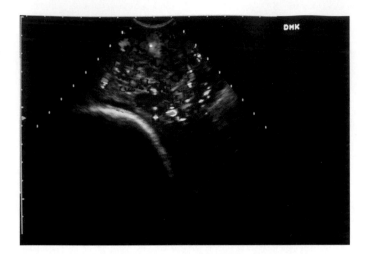

Chapter 12

Transvaginal Color Doppler Sonography

Arthur C. Fleischer, MD
Bhaskara K. Rao, MD
Donna M. Kepple, RDMS

Introduction

Color Doppler sonography (CDS) is a recent technological innovation that allows real-time sonographic visualization and evaluation of vascular structures both within and surrounding organs. This imaging capability has only recently been incorporated into a transvaginal probe. This configuration affords detailed delineation of the vasculature within and around the uterus and ovaries.

Since this technology is so new, there are only a few medical centers that have extensive experience with this technique. They include groups at the Kings College in London, the University of Zagreb in Yugoslavia, and our institution, Vanderbilt University. This chapter will cover our preliminary experience of this institution and that of these few other centers around the world, emphasizing the clinical applications of this technique for evaluating the uterus and ovaries.

Normal Anatomy and Scanning Technique

CDS, or color flow mapping, combines the physiologic information obtained by Doppler assessment of vessels with anatomic depiction of the location of blood flow within or adjacent to a particular organ. CDS assigns a color to the frequency shift detected; red colors indicate flow toward the transducer, whereas blue indicates flow away from the transducer. Lighter shades of color indicate high frequencies usually found in areas of stenosis.

The information obtained can be processed to form a triplex image consisting of a real-time image, color blood flow information, and a frequency waveform and spectral analysis displayed simultaneously. A disadvantage to this triplex format is that it requires relatively slow frame rates (4 to 6/sec), to acquire all the necessary information. The spectral information can be improved by freezing the image while obtaining the frequency spectra.

The information obtained on a waveform can be analyzed and quantitated in a variety of ways. Basically, the amount of parenchymal flow is reflected in the size and shape of the diastolic portion of the waveform. The frequencies contained in a waveform can be quantitated using either calculation of a resistive index (RI) or pulsatility index (PI). The PI is preferred, since it is more representative of the frequencies within the waveform, particularly when there are frequencies below the baseline. A PI is calculated by the computer program within the system by setting the cursor on the systolic peak then tracing it over the various frequencies to the end diastolic velocity. The system calculates a mean frequency and displays this on the monitor. The RI can be calculated by the systolic peak minus the end diastolic velocity divided by the systolic peak. RIs vary from 1.0 to 0, with 1.0 indicating the greatest resistance to forward flow. PIs typically range from 10.0 to 0. Basically, when there is increased diastolic velocities relative to systolic, the PI is low. Low PIs are typically seen within tumors since these masses have increased diastolic flow.

The intensities used for transvaginal (TV) CDS range from 52 to 60 mW/cm² spatial peak temporal average (SPTA), which is below the limit currently suggested by the Food and Drug Administration. The use of pulsed Doppler with color Doppler increases the intensities to 70 to 80 mW/cm².

Transvaginal CDS is performed using scanning maneuvers similar to those used for conventional transvaginal imaging. By color Doppler representation of vessels, one can maximize the clarity of the waveform received by moving the field of view so that the angle between the vessel and the incident beam is between 30 and 60 degrees.

The vascular anatomy of the pelvis is relatively constant with some variation in the size and flow of vessels depending on the parity status of the individual and whether or not previous surgeries have occurred.

The uterine artery is a branch of the hypogastric artery. As it courses toward the area of the cervix, it branches into an ascending branch coursing along the lateral aspects of the uterine corpus, and a descending branch coursing toward the cervix and upper vagina (Fig. 12-1). The ascending branch of the uterine artery is a relatively convoluted and tortuous vessel, and this should be taken into account when one assesses blood flow since it is normal to have both forward and reversed direction blood flow (below and above the spectral baseline) in a convoluted vessel. As the ascending branch of the uterine artery courses toward the cornu, there is an adnexal branch that continues to supply the ovary. The intramyometrial branches of the uterine artery form an arcuate configuration. Larger vessels course along the outer third of the myometrium and give off branches called radial arteries, which course in a spoke wheel pattern toward the endometrium. In general, the venous circulation of the uterus parallels the arterial. In the postmenopausal uterus, these vessels may be difficult to delineate because of their slow and relatively scant flow.

The ovary is supplied by two major arterial circulations; one from the adnexal branch of the uterine artery, the other from an ovarian artery that is a direct branch from the abdominal aorta (Fig. 12-2). The gonadal branch, which branches directly off the aorta, enters the area of the pelvis through the infindibulopelvic ligament along the lateral aspect of the ovary.

Other uterine and adnexal branches that may be occasionally seen are dilated vessels representing adnexal veins. The tubal arteries are rarely seen.

The typical arterial and venous velocities encountered in the utero-ovarian circulation range from 2 to 5 cm/sec. It has been shown with pulsed Doppler transvaginal sonography that the PI of the uterine and ovarian varies throughout the menstrual cycle with a gradual increase to the midcycle and a drop-off in the secretory phase (Scholtes et al, 1989). Typical PIs in normal uterine and ovarian vessels range between 3 and 4. A recently published study that used TV CDS for study of the uterine arteries showed a more complex temporal relationship between uterine blood flow ovarian morphology, and plasma concentrations of estradiol and progesterone. Peaks for the PI were observed on day 1 of menses, the day of plasma estradiol peak, and day of luteinizing hormone (LH) peak +3. Lowest PIs occurred on day of LH peak −6 and day of LH +9. Thus the highest PIs are found around the time of menses, with the lowest PI in the early follicular phase and subsequently during peak luteal function (Steer et al, 1990).

Uterine Disorders

CDS has the potential for assessment of uterine perfusion (Fig. 12-3). This can be obtained by measurement of velocities within the arcuate vessels. As in most organs, there is a gradual increase in the resistive index as one courses more distally from the main branches (Hata et al, 1989). Thus, the RIs encountered in the arcuate vessels are usually greater than that in the main uterine vessels.

One study has shown that duplex Doppler sonography can be helpful in assessing uterine perfusion in patients with failure to conceive during and after in vitro fertilization protocols. In this study, which used transabdominal duplex Doppler sonography, an increase in conception rate was documented after uterine perfusion was improved with oral administration of estrogens (Goswamy et al, 1988).

Other areas for evaluation of uterine perfusion with color Doppler imaging may include assessment of treatment in patients with choriocarcinoma or other invasive uterine tumors. We have documented a decrease in perfusion in a patient with a cervical ectopic treated with methotrexate (Fleischer et al, 1990) (Fig. 12-3A to E). Demonstration of choriodecidual vessels helps distinguish a pregnancy within a bicornuate uterus from a cornual ectopic pregnancy (Fig. 12-3F).

It is also possible that by delineation of the normal uterine vasculature, invasive tumors may be assessed to a greater degree of accuracy since the arcuate vessels typically delineate the outer two thirds of junction of the myometrium. CDS may also be helpful in diagnosis of carcinoma versus hyperplasia in that most tumors will demonstrate neovascularity. In a recently reported series the PI of the uterine arteries in cases of endometrial cancer was significantly lower than in women with bleeding not associated with cancer (Bourne et al, 1990).

Ovarian Disorders

CDS seems to have the potential for distinguishing benign from malignant ovarian tumors (Bourne et al, 1989) (Fig. 12-4). This distinction is based on detection of vessels that have high diastolic flow or low resistance, a common feature of vessels within tumors. As opposed to typical vessels that have a muscular intima, neovascular vessels typically lack this muscular coating and have numerous arteriovenous shunts. Both of these factors contribute to increased diastolic flow, which is apparent on the Doppler frequency waveform. In one study most malignant masses had PIs in the range of 0.3 to 1.0, whereas normal ovaries had PIs in the range of 3.1 to 9.4. In addition, malignant tumors demonstrated neovascularity that on CDS appeared as persistent and increased diastolic flow. Metabolically active benign tumors, such as dermoids containing thyroid cells or immature teratomas, may also mimic this pattern; however, we have also encountered some tumors that incited an extensive vascular reaction with low pulsatility indices.

A study performed by Kurjak and associates that included 151 patients with adnexal masses also showed high specificity and sensitivity of TV CDS in distinguishing benign from malignant ovarian masses. Using the resistivity index, all malignant masses had an RI less than 0.5 (Kurjak et al, 1990).

More extensive experience with this technique is required before one can assess its accuracy in distinguishing benign from malignant ovarian tumors. It does appear to have a potential role in distinguishing those ovarian masses that may be observed from those that need surgical excision.

Another major application of CDS using a transvaginal probe is in the detection of ovarian torsion. Ovarian torsion typically occurs when there has been significant hemorrhage into the ovary and a mass is present. Exaggerated folliculogenesis can precipitate the ovarian torsion (Figs. 12-5, 12-6). Early in the process there is venous and lymphatic obstruction, followed by arterial occlusion. In our limited experience, ovarian torsion appeared sonographically in enlarged ovaries that had no documentable perfusion in the parenchyma. It is possible that ovarian torsion might affect only one arterial supply to the ovary, and thus demonstrate partial perfusion. Even these ovaries should be surgically detorsed when one takes into account the intermittent nature of ovarian torsion.

Other Disorders

TV CDS can assess the myometrial vascularity associated with first trimester pregnancies. This has implications in distinguishing a cornual ectopic pregnancy from a normal pregnancy within a bicornuate or septated uterus, for example. It may also be helpful in establishing the intactness of the choriodecidua in an early pregnancy that is complicated by bleeding.

TV CDS can confirm the presence of markedly dilated pelvic vessels in patients with the clinically described pelvic congestion syndrome. This disorder has been described in multiparous women who have markedly dilated vessels that may contribute to pelvic pain, particularly when the patient stands or is postcoital. The pain can be precipitated by palpation over the ovaries (Beard et al, 1988). In this disorder, markedly dilated vessels (over 1 cm) can be seen with TV CDS with relatively slow flow (less than 2 to 3 cm/sec).

TV-CDS may be helpful in the diagnosis of placenta accreta. In this condition there is vascular involvement of the myometrium, which can be documented with TV CDS (Fig. 12-7).

Summary

This chapter discusses and illustrates preliminary experience with the application of TV CDS for evaluation of the uterus and ovaries. The main indications for this type of sonography include evaluation for ovarian torsion, distinguishing benign from malignant pelvic masses, diagnosis of pelvic congestion, and assessment of uteroovarian perfusion. Future applications will arise from active investigation with this new technique.

References

Beard RW, Reginald PW, Wadsworth J. Clinical features of women with chronic lower abdominal pain and pelvic congestion. *Br J Obstet Gynaecol* 1988;95:153–161.

Bourne T, Campbell S, Steer C, Whitehead MI, Collins WP. Transvaginal colour flow imaging: a possible new screening technique for ovarian cancer. *Br Med J* 1989;299:1367–1370.

Bourne T, Campbell S, Whitehead MI, Royston P, Steer CV, Collins WP. Detection of endometrial cancer in postmenopausal women by transvaginal ultrasonography and colour flow imaging. *Br Med J* 1990;301:18–25.

Fleischer AC, Rao BK, Kepple DM. Transvaginal color Doppler sonography: preliminary experiences. *Dynamic Cardiovasc Imaging*, 1990;3:52.

Goswamy RK, Williams G, Steptoe PC. Decreased uterine perfusion—a cause of infertility. *Hum Repro* 1988;3:955–959.

Hata T, Hata K, Senoh D, et al. Transvaginal Doppler color flow mapping. *Gynecol Obstet Invest* 1989;27:217–218.

Kurjak A, Zalud I, Alfirevic Z, Jurkovic D. The assessment of abnormal pelvic blood flow by transvaginal color and pulsed Doppler. *Ultrasound Med Biol* 1990;16:437–442.

Scholtes MCW, Wladimiroff JW, van Rijen HJM, Hop WCJ. Uterine and ovarian flow velocity waveforms in the normal menstrual cycle: a transvaginal Doppler study. *Fertil Steril* 1989;52:981–985.

Steer CV, Campbell S, Pampiglione JS, Kingsland CR, Mason BA, Collins WP. Transvaginal colour flow imaging of the uterine arteries during the ovarian and menstrual cycles. *Hum Repro* 1990;5:391–395.

Chapter *13*

Transperineal Scanning

Patricia C. Freeman, RT, RDMS
Philippe Jeanty, MD, PhD

Introduction

Adequate delineation of the cervix is a necessary part of every obstetric or gynecologic sonographic study. Obstetric patients who have third trimester bleeding need to have the region of the internal os evaluated for placenta previa, yet many physicians are wary of introducing a transvaginal transducer into the vagina in these patients. Transabdominal scans often fail to give the details necessary to rule out a placenta previa. The patient with an incompetent cervix also poses a diagnostic problem. Transperineal scanning can help in the evaluation of cervical abnormalities. First described in 1986, the transperineal scan has added a new diagnostic dimension to sonographic imaging of the cervical region (Jeanty et al, 1986).

Technique

Only minimal preparation of the transducer is necessary to perform a transperineal scan. A small amount of coupling gel is placed in a commercially available condom. The transducer is placed in the condom, and air bubbles are squeezed away from the face of the transducer. If necessary, a rubber band may be used to secure the condom around the neck of the transducer (Fig. 13-1*A*, *B*).

To perform a transperineal scan, the patient is positioned in the lithotomy position with legs bent and adducted (frog position). If the examination table has stirrups, they should be used to support the patient's legs. It is not necessary during perineal scans for the patient to have a full bladder. Ultrasonic gel is liberally applied directly to the vestibule between the labia. Care must be taken not to place the gel on the pubic hair, which would trap air bubbles. The transducer is placed directly on the vestibule with the probe directed in a sagittal orientation. Better contact is obtained by placing

the coupling gel directly on the patient rather than the probe since the gel is lost going through the pubic hair.

The orientation for this procedure is different from transabdominal scanning, and is the same as for transvaginal scanning. The equipment provides a right-to-left and top-to-bottom reversal switch to correct the orientation of the image, but the machine cannot perform a 90° rotation. The urinary bladder appears in the upper left position of the screen. The patient's feet are at the top of the screen and head at the bottom of the screen. Anterior is toward the left of the screen, and posterior to the right.

Normal Anatomy

To comprehend the new orientation of a transperineal scan, it is imperative to understand the normal anatomy (Fig. 13-2).

The pubic bone is in the upper left hand corner of the image. If a true sagittal scan is taken, the transducer beam passes through the symphysis pubis. Since the symphysis pubis is composed of fibrocartilage and hyaline cartilage, the ultrasound beam can readily pass through. If the transducer is on the bone instead, acoustic shadowing results, greatly degrading the image.

Directly below the pubic bone, an echo-free area is seen. This is the urinary bladder. Its size varies depending on the amount of urine present in the bladder at the time of the examination. Preferably the bladder is almost empty, because a distended bladder displaces the area of interest out of the image. The urethra appears as a hypoechoic tract that exits the bladder toward the perineum at the top of the image.

The vagina is located to the right of the symphysis and urethra. Like the urethra, it is a vertical hypoechoic structure. The hypoechoic portion corresponds to the muscular layer of the vaginal wall. The lumen is echogenic. If at all possible, it is advisable not to perform a

276

pelvic exam before the transperineal scan since a pelvic examination introduces air that will be trapped in the rugae of the vaginal canal. That air will cause shadowing, resulting in a suboptimal scan.

To the right (posterior) of the vagina is the rectum. The rectum may be filled with a variety of echo patterns depending on its contents.

The cervix is below the vagina, facing the urinary bladder or the transducer. It is recognizable by the typical trenchmouth appearance described by the French anatomist Rouviere. The endocervical canal is seen as a thin, echogenic line. A rounded, hypoechoic area can be seen to each side of the canal, joining the isthmus of the uterus.

Only the isthmus of the uterus and cervix can be identified. When information regarding the body or fundus of the uterus is needed, a transabdominal or transvaginal scan should be performed.

Indications for a Transperineal Scan

The transperineal scan is a useful adjunct to the transabdominal scan. It is most beneficial when viewing the cervix, lower uterine segment, or a retroflexed uterus. Transabdominal scans are better when the fundus of the uterus needs to be evaluated. Transvaginal sonography is excellent for examining the lower uterine segment, adnexa, or early pregnancy, but visualization and orientation of the cervix can be difficult. Each of these three scanning methods has its place in the imaging of the cervical region.

Several clinical problems may be solved by using the transperineal scan.

Incompetent cervix during pregnancy has proven to be a difficult diagnosis to make. Figure 13-3A demonstrates the transabdominal scan on a patient with an incompetent cervix. The cervix cannot be clearly seen. Figure 13-3B is the transperineal scan on the same patient. The dilated proximal endocervical canal can now be clearly seen with a cerclage suture in place. Figure 13-3C is the same patient 7 weeks later. Again, the dilated cervix with the cerclage suture in place is noted. Figure 13-4 demonstrates an incompetent cervix on transperineal scanning that was not apparent on transabdominal scanning. The reader is also referred to Chapter 10, which describes the appearance of cervical incompetence with transvaginal scanning.

Placenta previa can be difficult to rule out if the fetal head shadows the lower uterine segment. Figures 13-5 and 6 are transperineal scans performed to rule out placenta previa. In Fig. 13-6 the fetal head is shown to be snug against the internal os with no placenta previa.

At times the transabdominal sonogram (Fig. 13-7A) cannot delineate the margin of the placenta. A transperineal scan (Fig. 13-7B) demonstrates a space of 2.4 cm between the inferior edge of the placenta and the internal os, excluding the diagnosis of placenta previa. Figure 13-8 is an example of a transperineal scan performed on a patient with a complete placenta previa. The internal os is completely covered by the placenta.

An early intrauterine pregnancy in a retroflexed uterus can be difficult to delineate transabdominally, and documenting fetal heart motion may be impossible because of the attenuation of the sound beam. If a transvaginal transducer is not available, a transperineal scan should be performed. Figure 13-9 is an example of a transperineal scan in a patient with a retroflexed uterus demonstrating the gestational sac, fetus, and fetal heart motion.

Urinary stress incontinence had previously been diagnosed by either the cystourethrogram or a bead-chain cystogram. Genuine urinary stress incontinence in women is associated with a downward and posterior rotational descent of the urethrovesical junction. The increase in intra-abdominal pressure transmitted to the outside of the bladder is then no longer transmitted to the urethra, and urine loss results (Korhorn et al, 1986). Surgery is more beneficial if the anatomic defect can be visualized. A transperineal scan to demonstrate the bladder neck and urethra allows all the information previously provided by radiography to be visualized without radiation, catheters, or bead-chains. The transperineal scan for urinary stress incontinence is performed exactly as described previously.

Cervical evaluation is difficult in young girls who are still virgins. A transabdominal scan may not provide the necessary information, and the transvaginal transducer is not an option because of their virginity. Figure 13-10 is a transperineal scan of a 14-year-old virgin. The patient's transabdominal scan revealed some echoes in her cervix of questionable cause. A transperineal scan was performed to better evaluate those echoes. Air bubbles were visualized throughout the vaginal canal. A repeat transperineal scan 1 week later failed to demonstrate any bubbles.

Vaginal atresia has recently been evaluated with transperineal scanning. In patients with hydro/hematocolpos whose obstruction is low lying, transperineal scans can best identify the level of the obstruction and the thickness of the obstructing septum. The study for vaginal atresia is performed with a standoff pad to allow for improved imaging of the superficial structures and a more accurate measurement of the distance from the perineum to the caudal margin of the distended vagina. Once the greatest caudal extension has been ascertained in the sagittal plane, the transducer is rotated to the coronal position. The distance from the perineum to the caudal aspect of the distended vagina is then measured to aid in decisions concerning the surgical reconstruction (Scanlan et al, 1990).

Summary

The transperineal scan is a useful supplement to the transabdominal scan. It is easy to perform, does not require an additional transducer (making the exam cost-efficient), and can be used on young women who are still virgins. Because no transducer is introduced into the vagina, it can be used to assess vaginal bleeding associated with placenta previa. By measuring the urethral angle, information can be obtained for the diagnosis of urinary stress incontinence. Therefore,

when additional information is needed pertaining to the cervical area, a transperineal scan should be performed (Fig. 13-11).

References

Jeanty P, d'Altan M, Romero R, Hobbins J. Perineal scanning. *Am J Perinatol* 1986;3:289–295.

Korhorn E, Scioscia A, Jeanty P, Hobbins J. Ultrasound cystourethrography by perineal scanning for the assessment of female stress urinary incontinence. *Obstet Gynecol* 1986;68:269–272.

Scanlan K, Pozniak M, Fagerholm M, Shapiro S. Value of transperineal sonography in the assessment of vaginal atresia. *AJR* 1990;154:545–548.

FIGURE 13-1 *A.* Materials needed to perform a transperineal scan. *B.* Transducer prepared for a transperineal scan.

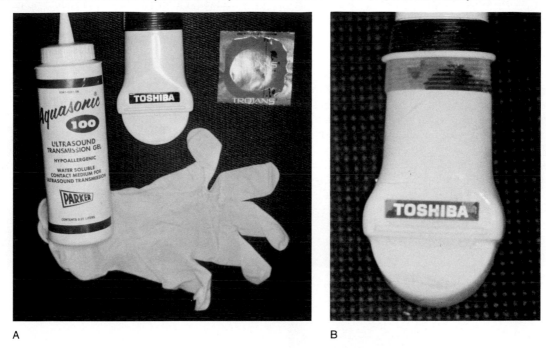

A   B

FIGURE 13-2 Orientation for a transperineal scan. Caudal is at the top of the image and cranial is at the bottom. Anterior is to the left of the image and posterior to the right. B, bladder; VC, vaginal canal; R, rectum; CX, cervix; arrow, endocervical canal; curved arrow, urethra. (Reproduced with permission from Jeanty, Romero. *Obstetrical Ultrasound.* In preparation.)

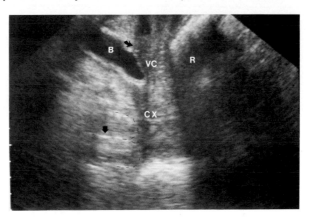

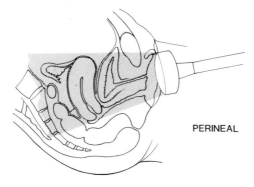

PERINEAL

FIGURE 13-3   *A.* Transabdominal scan on a patient with incompetent cervix. The curved arrow points at the cervix, which is not well evaluated. B, maternal bladder; F, fetus. *B.* Transperineal scan on the same patient as in *A* demonstrating a dilated endocervical canal (C) with a cerclage suture in place (arrows). *C.* Same patient 7 weeks later. Again note the dilated endocervical canal with the cerclage sutures. (Reproduced with permission from Jeanty, Romero. *Obstetrical Ultrasound.* In preparation.)

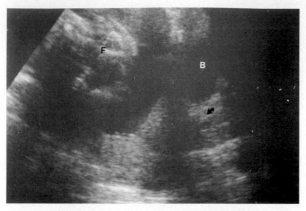

A

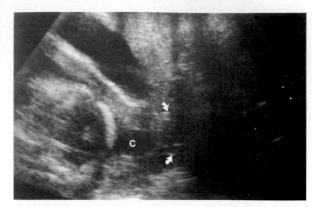

B

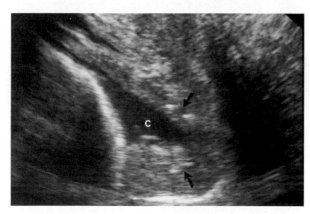

C

FIGURE 13-4 **Incompetent Cervix.** *A*. Transabdominal sonogram shows a normal cervix. *B*. Transperineal scan shows definite dilation of the endocervical canal.

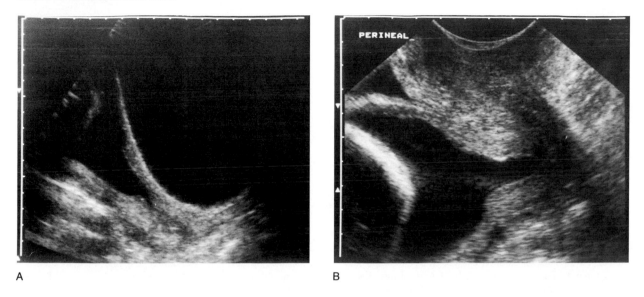

A   B

FIGURE 13-5 **Complete Placenta Previa.** *A*. Transabdominal sonogram showing posterior placenta extending into area of internal cervical os. *B*. Transperineal scan confirming a complete previa. The urinary bladder is moderately distended.

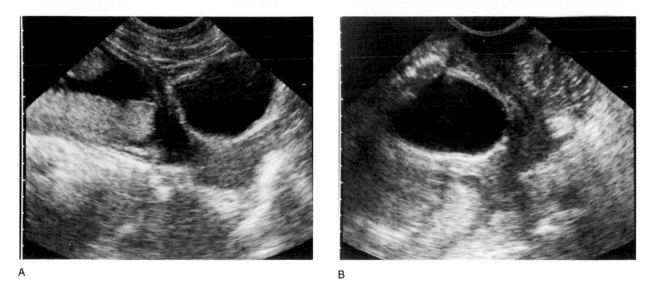

A   B

FIGURE 13-6   Transperineal scan to rule out placenta previa. The fetal head (F) is snug against the internal os (IO) with no evidence of placenta previa. (Reproduced with permission from Jeanty, Romero. *Obstetrical Ultrasound*. In preparation.)

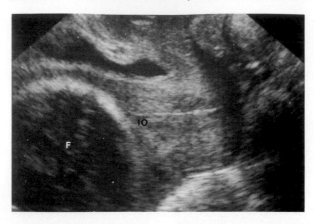

FIGURE 13-7   *A.* Longitudinal midline transabdominal scan to rule out placenta previa. Placental edge cannot be deliniated from myometrium. *B.* The transperineal scan of the same patient demonstrates a space of 2.4 cm between the placenta (P) and internal os of the cervix (C), thereby excluding placenta previa. (Reproduced with permission from Jeanty, Romero. *Obstetrical Ultrasound*. In preparation.)

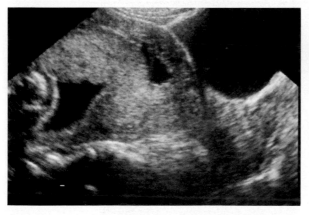 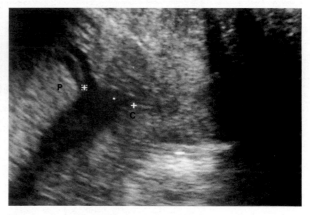

A   B

FIGURE 13-8 Transperineal scan on a patient with a complete placenta previa. B, bladder; P, placenta; IO, internal os. (Reproduced with permission from Jeanty, Romero. *Obstetrical Ultrasound*. In preparation.)

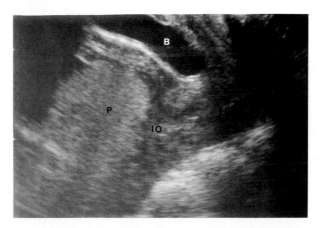

FIGURE 13-9 Transperineal scan of 12-week intrauterine pregnancy with fetal heart motion documented on M-mode.

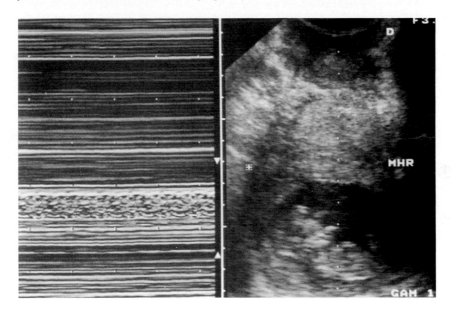

FIGURE 13-10 Transperineal scan in 14-year-old virgin showing echoes within the vagina (arrows) probably arising from trapped air after a pelvic exam.

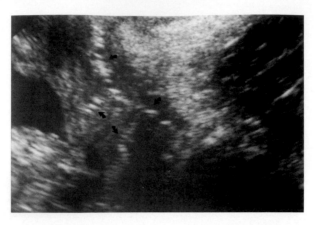

FIGURE 13-11 Transperineal scan of a patient with a cervical pregnancy. Transvaginal sonography gave the most information and transabdominal the least. When transvaginal sonography is not available, transperineal scanning should be the method of choice to evaluate the cervical region. SP, symphysis pubis; VC, vaginal canal; R, rectum; U, uterus; CP, cervical pregnancy. (Reproduced with permission from Jeanty, Romero. *Obstetrical Ultrasound*. In preparation.)

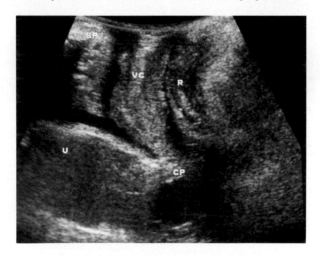

Chapter 14

Transrectal Sonography

Arthur C. Fleischer, MD

Introduction

Transrectal sonography can be used in several gynecologic conditions. The same probe used for prostate imaging in men can be applied for visualization of the uterus and adnexal regions and cul-de-sac in women. Although the transrectal approach is not as close to the uterus as transvaginal scanning, it allows the sonographer to have unencumbered access to the vagina for certain intraoperative procedures. Thus, the main applications of this type of scanning are for intraoperative guidance, for difficult dilation and curettage procedures when there is an abnormal cervix, for localization of the cervix for tandem placement for intracavitary radiation when there are cervical abnormalities, for extraction of intrauterine contraceptive devices that may be difficult to retrieve, and for guidance for cerclage in abnormal cervices. Additionally, it may be useful in the evaluation of patients with suspected cystocele or enterocele or lower urinary tract disorder.

Instrumentation and Scanning Techniques

There are several types of transrectal probes. These include probes that have biplane imaging capabilities (sagittal and axial) and those probes that use a single element transducer that is rotated in a radial fashion (Fig. 14-1). The biplane probe is preferred for intraoperative guidance of intrauterine procedures. Initially the cervix is located in its long axis with the longitudinally oriented linear array transducer. The field of view can be confirmed on an image obtained with the axial transducer typically located at the end of the probe.

As opposed to transducer-probe preparation for the transvaginal probe, the transrectal probe has only water placed between the probe and the condom interface. Then fluid within the condom (20 to 33 mL) surrounding the transducer provides adequate transmission through the condom and into the area of interest. Gel is applied to the outer surface of the condom to provide optimal through transmission through the rectal wall.

When the biplane probe is used intraoperatively, one should be aware that metal objects such as retractors will block the ultrasound transmission. Therefore the smallest retractor possible must be held out of the plane of the incident beam for adequate delineation of the uterus.

Normal Anatomy

As imaged in the long axis on transrectal sonography, the uterus appears as a pear-shaped structure. Typically the mucous within the endocervical canal appears as an angled echogenic interface with the remainder of the endometrium being thicker than the endocervical canal (Fig. 14-2). On axial images, the cervix appears as a rounded structure with a central echogenic area representing the endocervical canal. Usually the adnexal regions appear as moderately echogenic areas with no significant soft tissue intervening between bowel and the rectal wall.

Because of the proximity of the transrectal probe to the cervix, it is not uncommon to see small (2 to 3 mm), well-defined hypoechoic structures near the endocervical canal that represent distended endocervical glands. Nabothian cysts can also be demonstrated as cystic structures in this region, but are usually larger than 5 mm. Along the lateral aspects of the upper cervix, punctate hypoechoic structures can be demonstrated that represent the perforating branches of the uterine artery. These vessels usually enter the myometrium at the level of the internal cervical os and can serve as a landmark for this region of the uterus.

Intraoperative Guidance

Transrectal sonography is helpful in difficult cases where the cervical os may not be apparent to the operator on visual inspection (Fleischer et al, 1990). Such cases occur when there is cervical stenosis, cervical carcinoma, or a malformed cervix (Figs. 14-3, 14-4). Scanning through the transrectal approach allows the operator to manipulate instrumentation vaginally.

This approach can be used for initial localization of the cervix before dilation and curettage. It can also be used to locate the cervical lumen when an intrauterine tandem is required before intracavitary radiation (Fig. 14-5). This technique has also been used in localizing the cervical tissue for cerclage, particularly in patients who have had previous conization (Fleischer et al, 1989) (Figs. 14-6, 14-7).

Diagnosis of Cystocele and Enterocele

Transrectal sonography can be used for diagnosis and differentiation of cystocele from rectocele. Cystoceles appear as cystic structures contiguous with the bladder lumen (Fig. 14-8). The structure usually enlarges and protrudes inferiorly when the patient strains. Enteroceles appear as echogenic structures that lie between the bladder and the rectum.

Other Applications

Transrectal sonography has been used for evaluation of patients with stress urinary incontinence (Bergman et al, 1988). The advantage of this technique over transperineal scanning is that the area is not deformed by the pressure from the transducer itself. Criteria have been established for abnormal displacement of the urethra, as documented by a change in the interface arising from a Q-tip in the urethra. Abnormal angulation and motility of over 1.5 cm has been defined as abnormal, indicative of stress urinary incontinence (Bergman et al, 1988). Some investigators have used transrectal sonography for diagnosis of recurrence of ovarian and uterine neoplasms (Squillaci et al, 1988). With recurrent tumor, hypoechoic masses in the region of the vaginal cuff have been described.

Using the radially oriented probe, some have evaluated the anus for perianal abscesses and fistula. Using this technique, disruptions in the typical five-layered interface appearance arising from the colon in the area of the internal sphincter can be identified (Law et al, 1989). Intersphincteric abscesses, retained, or foreign material such as sutures and other abnormalities surrounding the anus can be identified using this technique.

Summary

This chapter describes the application of transrectal sonography for a variety of gynecologic disorders. It is most useful in intraoperative guidance, but can also be used for diagnosis of enterocele and cystocele.

References

Bergman A, Vermesh R, Platt I. Ultrasonic evaluation of UVJ in women with stress urinary incontinence. *J Clin Ultrasound* 1988;16:295–300.

Fleischer A, Burnett L, Jones H, Murphy M. Transrectal sonography for guidance of intraoperative uterine procedures. *Radiology* 1990;176:576–577.

Fleischer A, Lombardi S, Kepple D. Transrectal sonography for guidance during cerclage. *J Ultrasound Med* 1989;8:589–591.

Law P, Talbot R, Bartram C. Anal endosonography in the evaluation of perianal sepsis and fistula *in ano. Br J Surg* 1989;76:752–755.

Squillaci E, Salzani M, Grandinetti M, Auffermann W. Recurrence of ovarian and uterine neoplasms: diagnosis with transrectal US. *Radiology* 1988;169:355–358.

FIGURE 14-1 Diagram of imaging planes obtained by biplane transrectal transducer-probe. The longitudinally oriented linear array images in the sagittal plane whereas the axially oriented curvilinear array at the tip of the probe images in the axial plane.

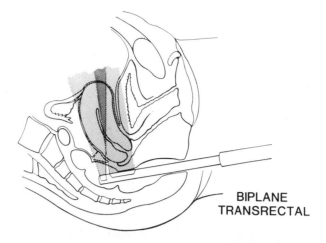

BIPLANE
TRANSRECTAL

FIGURE 14-2 *A*. Normal uterus shown from transrectal approach. *B*. The endometrial thickness is measured by cursors.

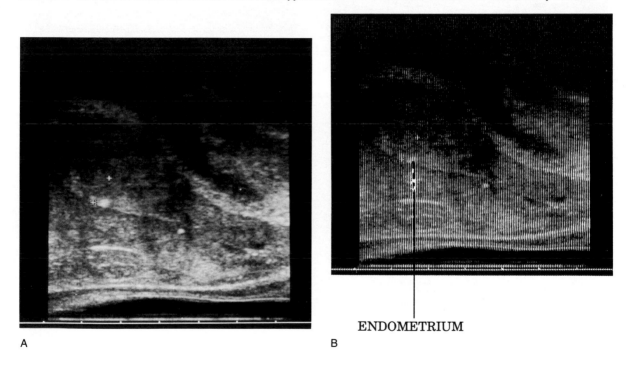

ENDOMETRIUM

A   B

FIGURE 14-3   It was initially difficult to cannulate the cervical os in a patient with thickened endometrium and postmenopausal bleeding. Transrectal sonography provided guidance for dilatation and curettage.

14-3A   Transrectal sagittal scan shows thickened endometrium in an anteflexed uterus.

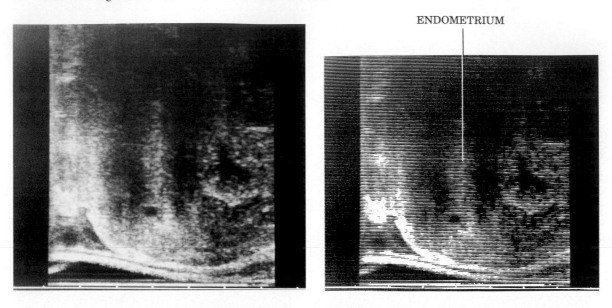

14-3B   Initial attempts to pass the dilator were unsuccessful because the dilator was directed posteriorly.

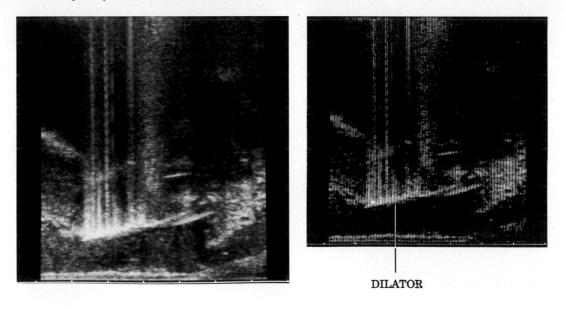

(continued)

FIGURE 14-3 It was initially difficult to cannulate the cervical os in a patient with thickened endometrium and postmenopausal bleeding. Transrectal sonography provided guidance for dilatation and curettage. *(continued)*

14-3C With more anterior direction of the dilator, the cervical canal was successfully entered and endometrium curetted. A mildly distended bladder coupled with posterior pressure on the rectum by the condom-covered probe helped straighten out the uterus to facilitate curettage.

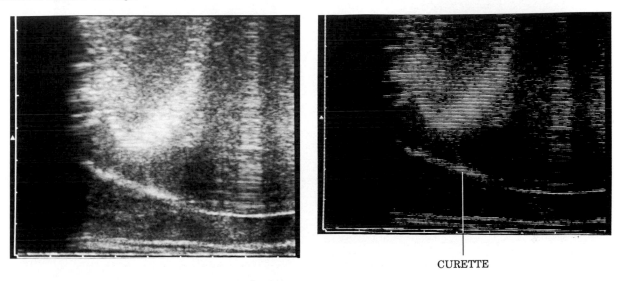

CURETTE

FIGURE 14-4 Guidance Into a Blind-Ended Duplicated Cervix in a Patient Who Had Purulent Discharge

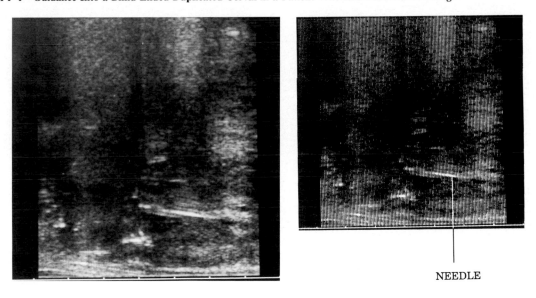

NEEDLE

FIGURE 14-5   **Guided Intrauterine Tandem Placement in a Patient with Extensive Cervical Carcinoma**

14-5A   The endocervical canal was localized in long (*A*) and short (*B*) axes.

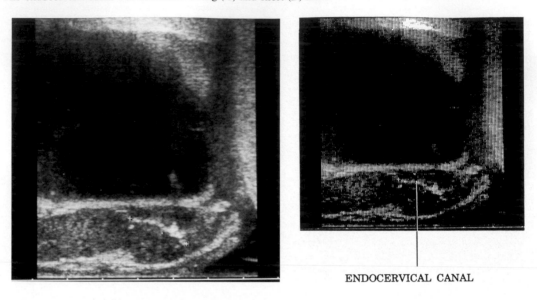

ENDOCERVICAL CANAL

14-5B   The endocervical canal was localized in long (*A*) and short (*B*) axes.

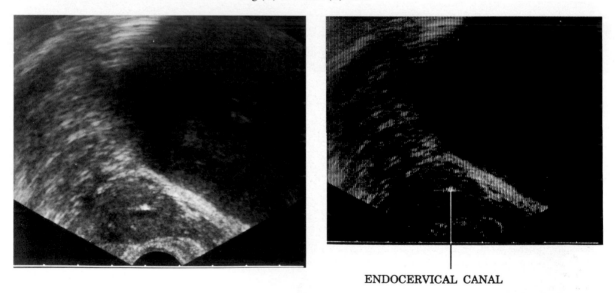

ENDOCERVICAL CANAL

(continued)

FIGURE 14-5   **Guided Intrauterine Tandem Placement in a Patient with Extensive Cervical Carcinoma** *(continued)*

14-5C   The tandem was subsequently introduced into the uterine lumen, as confirmed in long *(C)* and short *(D)* axes views.

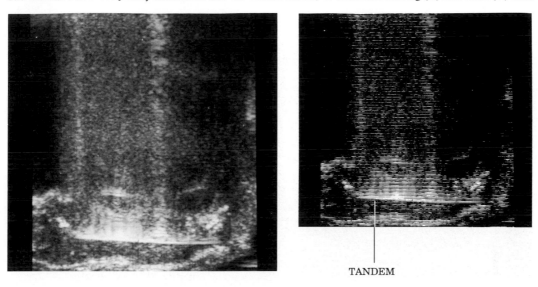

TANDEM

14-5D   The tandem was subsequently introduced into the uterine lumen, as confirmed in long *(C)* and short *(D)* axes views.

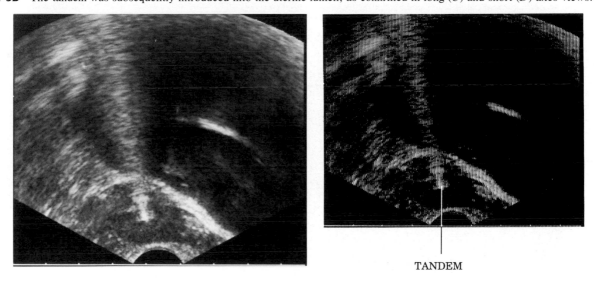

TANDEM

FIGURE 14-6   Cerclage Placement in a Patient Status after Three Conizations

14-6A   Initial transrectal sonogram shows a shortened (2.1 cm) cervix in long axis (between cursors)

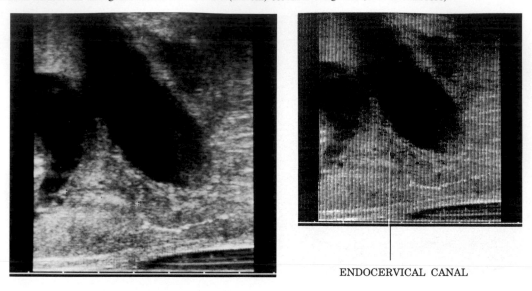

ENDOCERVICAL CANAL

14-6B   Suture in place around the endocervical canal, approximately 1 cm deep to external os as seen in long (*B*) and short axes. The circular course of the suture could be appreciated on the axial scan.

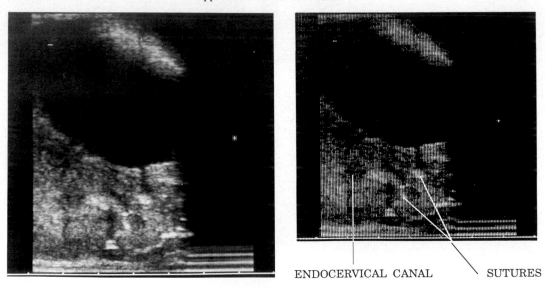

ENDOCERVICAL CANAL   SUTURES

FIGURE 14-7   Confirmation of Normal Cervix after Cerclage

14-7A   A nondistended endocervical canal is seen, as well as the suture within the lower posterior of the cervix.

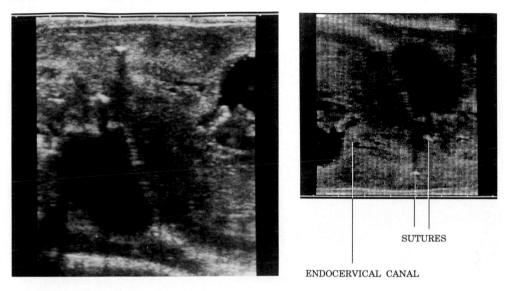

SUTURES

ENDOCERVICAL CANAL

14-7B   The circular shape of the suture is seen on an axial transrectal sonogram.

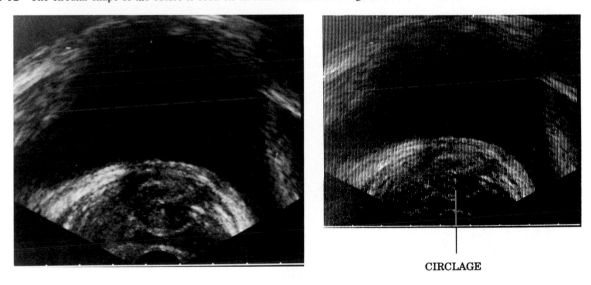

CIRCLAGE

FIGURE 14-8   **Transrectal Sonography of Cystocele**

14-8A   An ill-defined cystic structure is seen.

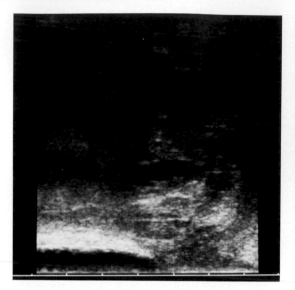
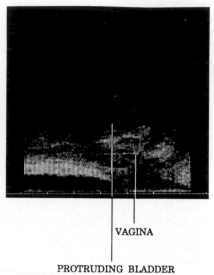

VAGINA

PROTRUDING BLADDER

14-8B   During straining the bladder protrudes into the perineum.

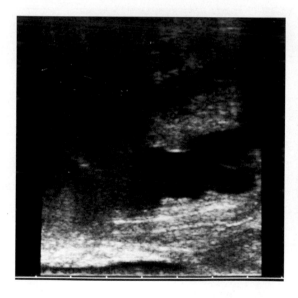
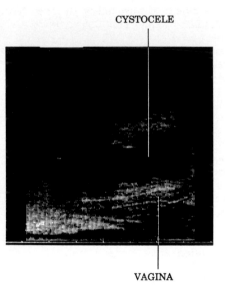

CYSTOCELE

VAGINA

Index

Page numbers in italics indicate figures; page numbers followed by a "t" indicate tables; figure numbers in boldface indicate figures in Chapter 12 color insert.